Infection in the Critically Ill: an Ongoing Challenge

Springer

Milano
Berlin
Heidelberg
New York
Barcelona
Hong Kong
London
Paris
Singapore
Tokyo

van Saene H.K.F.
Sganga G.
Silvestri L. (Eds)

Infection in the Critically Ill: an Ongoing Challenge

Series edited by
Antonino Gullo

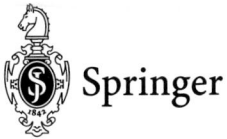 Springer

H.K.F. van Saene
Department of Clinical Microbiology/Infection Control
Royal Liverpool Children's NHS, Liverpool, UK

G. Sganga
Department of Surgery/Division of Organ Transplantation
Catholic University, University Hospital Agostino Gemelli and CNR
Centro Studi Fisiopatologia Shock, Rome, Italy

L. Silvestri
Department of Anaesthesia and Intensive Care
Gorizia Hospital, Gorizia, Italy

Series of *Topics in Anaesthesia and Critical Care* edited by
A. Gullo
Department of Clinical Science, Section of Anaesthesia, Intensive Care and
Pain Clinic
Cattinara Hospital, Trieste, Italy

Springer-Verlag Italia
a member of BertelsmannSpringer Science+Business Media GmbH

© Springer-Verlag Italia, Milano 2001

ISBN 88-470-0138-2

Cover design: Simona Colombo, Milan
Typesetting and layout: Photo Life, Vimodrone (Milan)
Printing and binding: Centro Grafico Ambrosiano, San Donato (Milan)
Printed in Italy

SPIN: 10789965

Foreword

Infections contracted by patients constitute an important factor in the management of any hospital unit. For patients with weakened resistance due to trauma, after surgery and in intensive care, infection-related complications have a negative impact on care quality indicators, specifically in terms of protracted hospitalisation time, increased costs from complications and extended hospitalisation, and increased mortality rate. Effective strategies to prevent and treat infections are a priority in optimising the cost-effectiveness of care. Infection control, diagnostics and targeted antibiotic therapy require an integrated epidemiological, microbiological and clinical approach. This is indispensable for critically ill patients, especially when the processes of infection and sepsis are supported by micro-organisms which are multidrug-resistant and difficult to root out.

The importance of this subject has been demonstrated by a European observational study on the prevalence of hospital infections in patients under intensive care. In this study, the prevalence of infections contracted in a "high-risk" environment was 21%, while other studies have observed that the incidence of pneumonia in patients undergoing artificial ventilation varied between 8% and 54%, with a median of 24%. These figures alone are enough to show the clinical importance of the infective process and the need for continuous interdisciplinary updating and exchanges of experience.

Great attention is currently being paid to the treatment of peritonitis and the prophylactic use of antibiotics in high-risk surgical patients. The translocation of bacteria is a subject that requires further research, since the extent of this process in clinical practice has yet to be fully established. The microbiology of patients being treated with selective decontamination of the digestive tract is another key subject. Although this technique is controversial, little used and in some respects highly criticised, evidence-base medicine has clearly proved its effectiveness. Techniques of culture monitoring, especially for gram-negative multidrug-resistant bacteria, is another interesting theme. The proper use of antibiotics for the treatment of methicillin-resistant staphylococcus infections is a topical subject in light of recent therapeutic advances. New methods for controlling *Acinetobacter* infections and problems related to drug resistance are dealt with fully in the specialised literature. It was decided in this volume to discuss only the features of the greatest clinical interest and relevance to research on infections. The aim was to provide concise updating for researchers, clinicians and specialists in the subject.

I am grateful to the colleagues who have supported this initiative and have contributed their expertise. My special thanks go to Rick van Saene, Gabriele Sganga and Luciano Silvestri for a number of reasons, especially for the enthusiasm and friendship they have unstintingly provided in the preparation of this important update and for their acknowledged leadership, which augurs well for the success of this new publishing initiative.

Antonino Gullo

Preface

"The essential of intensive care is the prevention of complications"

CP Stoutenbeek [1948-1998]

Infection in the critically ill is an on-going challenge. Rates of pneumonia and septicaemia have not changed since the inception of intensive care in the 1960s. One third of critically ill adults still die, most from their underlying disease, and resultant immuno-paralysis complicated by infection. However, forty years later we are in a worse position as practically all micro-organisms have exhibited varying degrees of resistance to even the most potent antibiotics. Currently we have no new classes of antibiotics available. Outbreaks of multi-resistant organisms are now common place in many intensive care units, and the public is increasingly aware of the risks of developing nosocomial infection whilst in hospital. Hence intensivists are searching for alternative approaches to managing infection on their ICU.

In the early 1980s, Dr CP Stoutenbeek advocated a different approach to the management of infection, that of a pre-emptive strike. He introduced a novel and controversial concept, which he termed selective decontamination of the digestive tract [SDD]. His ideas were based upon surveillance of the carrier state and use of prophylactic antibiotics both enteral and parenteral. Despite antagonism from various quarters and generalised ignorance leading to a negative attitude towards the practice, SDD still commands a high profile. The realisation that medical practice must be based upon evidence rather than expert opinion consummated in two recent meta-analyses of randomised SDD trials. They confirmed that Stoutenbeek's approach produced a significant reduction in morbidity and mortality, which stimulated a resurgence in the interest of SDD.

In this book we develop Stoutenbeek's original concept. It is based on the 14th APICE meeting in Trieste 1999 and describes how to prevent and treat pneumonia and septicaemia in critically ill patients. The studies presented show that the use of oral non-absorbable antimicrobials may prolong the antibiotic era. The work concludes by dealing with outbreak situations, both analysis and control.

Finally we dedicate this issue to the memory of Chris Stoutenbeek, an intensivist who was at heart an anaesthetist, he saw his vision of preventative intensive care develop into a sound evidence-based manoeuvre.

HKF van Saene, G Sganga, L Silvestri

Trieste, January 2001

Acknowledgements

The Editors wish to thank Dr. A. Torres, from the Clinical Institute of Pneumology and Thoracic Surgery, Barcelona, Spain, who provided the cover figure: pneumonia is a multi-focal process affecting both lungs primarily the lower lobes, supporting the technique of blind sampling (arrow) using tracheal aspirates as a good diagnostic utility.

Contents

Contributors

Álvarez M.
Intensive Care Unit, University Hospital Príncipe de Asturias, Madrid, Spain

Barrett S.P.
Department of Infection, Guy's Hospital, London, UK

Baines P.
Department of Paediatric Intensive Care, Royal Liverpool Children's NHS Trust of Alder Hey, Liverpool, UK

Bauer T.
Department of Pneumology and Respiratory Medicine, Hospital Clinic i Provincial, Barcelona, Spain

Bosman R.J.
Department of Intensive Care Medicine, OLVG, Amsterdam, The Netherlands

Brisinda G.
Department of Surgery, Division of Organ Transplantation, Catholic University, University Hospital Agostino Gemelli and CNR, Centro Studio Fisiopatologia Shock, Rome, Italy

Calderón M.
Department of Critical Care Medicine, Hospital Universitario de Getafe, Madrid, Spain

Castagneto M.
Department of Surgery, Division of Organ Transplantation, Catholic University, University Hospital Agostino Gemelli and CNR, Centro Studio Fisiopatologia Shock, Rome, Italy

Cerdá E.
Department of Critical Care Medicine, Hospital Universitario de Getafe, Madrid, Spain

Corbella X.
Infectious Disease Service, Hospital de Bellvitge, Barcelona, Spain

De Gaudio A.R.
Department of Medical, Surgical Critical Care, Section of Anesthesiology
and Intensive Care, University of Florence, Florence, Italy

de la Cal M.A.
Department of Critical Care Medicine, Hospital Universitario de Getafe,
Madrid, Spain

Ferrer R.
Department of Paediatric Intensive Care, Royal Liverpool Children's NHS Trust
of Alder Hey, Liverpool, UK

Fontana F.
Department of Laboratory Medicine and Microbiology, Presidio Ospedaliero,
Gorizia, Italy

French G.L.
Department of Microbiology, Guy's, King's & St Thomas' School of Medicine,
St Thomas' Hospital, London, UK

García-Hierro P.
Department of Medical Microbiology, Hospital Universitario de Getafe,
Madrid, Spain

Hughes J.
Department of Clinical Microbiology and Infection Control, Royal Liverpool
Children's NHS Trust of Alder Hey, Liverpool, UK

Meyer J.
University of California, Riverside University of Southern California,
Los Angels, USA

Petros A.J.
Department of Paediatric Anaesthesia and Intensive Care, Institute
of Child Health and Great Ormond Street, Hospital for Children NHS Trust,
London, UK

Reilly N.
Department of Pharmacy, Royal Liverpool Children's NHS Trust of Alder Hey,
Liverpool, UK

Sánchez M.
Intensive Care Unit, University Hospital Príncipe de Asturias, Madrid, Spain

Sarginson R.
Department of Paediatric Intensive Care, Royal Liverpool Children's NHS Trust
of Alder Hey, Liverpool, UK

Sganga G.
Department of Surgery, Division of Organ Transplantation, Catholic University,
University Hospital Agostino Gemelli and CNR, Centro Studio Fisiopatologia
Shock, Rome, Italy

Silvestri L.
Department of Anaesthesia and Intensive Care, Gorizia Hospital,
Gorizia, Italy

Sitges-Serra A.
Department of Surgery, Hospital Universitari del Mar, Barcelona, Spain

Shankar K.R.
Department of Paediatric Surgery, Royal Liverpool Children's NHS Trust
of Alder Hey, Liverpool, UK

Taylor N.
Department of Clinical Microbiology and Infection Control, Royal Liverpool
Children's NHS Trust of Alder Hey, Liverpool, UK

Toltzis P.
Division of Pharmacology and Critical Care, Department of Pediatrics, Case
Western Reserve University School of Medicine, Cleveland, USA

Torres A.
Clinical Institute of Pneumology and Thoracic Surgery, Hospital Clinic
i Provincial, Barcelona, Spain

van Saene H.K.F.
Department of Clinical Microbiology and Infection Control, Royal Liverpool
Children's NHS Trust of Alder Hey, Liverpool, UK

Zandstra D.F.
Department of Intensive Care Medicine, OLVG, Amsterdam, The Netherlands

Chapter 1

Pneumonia Management in the Intensive Care Unit: an Integrated Approach

D.F. ZANDSTRA, H.K.F. VAN SAENE, R.J. BOSMAN

Introduction

Treatment of pneumonia in the intensive care unit (ICU) includes two different entities: firstly, treatment of patients admitted with pneumonia which may be either community (CAP) or hospital acquired (HAP), and secondly, prevention/treatment of ventilator associated pneumonia (VAP).

Treatment of Community- and Hospital-Acquired Pneumonia Patients with Respiratory Insufficiency when Admitted to the Intensive Care Unit and Prevention of Ventilator-Associated Pneumonia

HAP necessitating ICU treatment with mechanical ventilation has a notoriously high mortality rate, ranging from 33% to 90%, and is difficult to treat. While patients remain intubated, it is difficult to eradicate aerobic gram-negative bacilli (AGNB) from the respiratory tract with systemic antibiotics alone, even using new potent antibiotics. The incidence of relapse and superinfection with multi-resistant strains is high.

The treatment of respiratory insufficiency in critically ill, mechanically ventilated patients is often complicated by the onset of pneumonia (VAP).

VAP contributes significantly to increased morbidity (length of stay, LOS) and increased mortality risk [1-5]. A few studies failed to confirm these data [6, 7].

It is clear from several meta-analysis studies that VAP can be significantly reduced by selective decontamination of the digestive tract (SDD) [8, 9]. In the management of CAP and HAP in the ICU, the prevention of complicating VAP and the cure rate have received only limited attention [10]. However, VAP is a well known complication of CAP and also increases mortality [11]. Initial treatment of HAP and CAP will be based on clinical judgement, since all forms of microbiological diagnostics require time. Timely institution of adequate antibiotic therapy in critical conditions reduces mortality and morbidity.

Although the clinical diagnosis of pneumonia is not difficult (fever/hypothermia, impaired function, purulent sputum, leucocytosis or leucopaenia), the choice of the initial antibiotic therapy remains difficult if no framework is present. The quickest available method of determining the type of micro-organisms involved is gram stain of the tracheal aspirate.

The aim of this chapter is to present a workframe to treat HAP and CAP and to prevent VAP, thus providing adequate strategies for succesful treatment and prevention. Within this workframe 11 important definitions should be familiar to the intensive care physician in order to understand the pathogenesis of pneumonia and to implement therapy and prevention [12]. Standardization of terms and definitions in the context of CAP, HAP and VAP is crucial to guarantee consistency [12].

Definitions

Potentially Pathogenic Micro-organisms

Potentially pathogenic micro-organisms (PPM) are micro-organisms with an intrinsic pathogenicity index (IPI), i.e. the ratio of infected patients to carriers of a particular pathogen, which lies between 0.1 and 0.3. The IPI is nearly 1 for *Salmonella* species, while micro-organism with a low intrinsic pathogenicity pathogens, including indigenous flora, have an IPI varying between 0.01-0.03.

PPM cause infection when the patient has impaired defence mechanisms. Community PPM (*Streptococcus pneumoniae, Haemophilius influenzae, Moraxella catarrhalis, Escherichia coli, Staphylococcus aureus* and *Candida* species) should be distinguished from hospital or opportunistic PPM (*Klebsiella, Proteus, Morganella, Enterobacter, Serratia, Acinetobacter* and *Pseudomonas* species).

In general, the six micro-organisms listed as community PPM cause infections in previously healthy patients, while the eight AGNB cause infection in patients with compromised defence mechanisms due to underlying disease.

The indigenous flora of the gut and skin does not fit into the definition of PPM because its intrinsic pathogenicity (IPI < 0.003) is very low.

Carriage

Carriage defines a state where the same strain of PPM is isolated from at least two consecutive surveillance samples (saliva, gastric juice, faeces, throat and rectal swabs) in any concentration over a period of 1 week. Acquisition carriage is considered to exist if a sample is positive for a PPM that differs from the previous isolates. Thus carriage is the persistent presence of micro-organisms, usually in the oropharynx and gut.

Colonisation

Colonisation is the presence of a PPM in an internal organ that is normally sterile (bladder, lower respiratory tract). The diagnostic sample reveals less than 100,000 colony forming units (CFU) per millilitre of diagnostic sample.

Bacterial Infection

Bacterial infection is a microbiologically proven clinical diagnosis. Apart from the clinical signs of infection, the diagnostic sample obtained contains more than 100.000 CFU per millilitre of sample or is positive in the case of blood.

Colonisation traditionally is distinguished from infection in order to reduce or restrict the use of antibiotics.

From the point of view of prevention of infection, infections in the ICU may be classified into three different categories:

1. Primary endogenous infections are caused by both community and hospital PPM that are carried by the patient on admission to the ICU, e.g. *S. aureus* pneumonia after intubation of a trauma patient or a post-surgical intra-abdominal infection caused by *Morganella morganii*.
2. Secondary endogenous infections are caused by PPM acquired after admission to the ICU. They invariably belong to the group of hospital-PPM, e.g. *Acinetobacter* pneumonia. After acquisition, carriage develops, followed by colonisation and infection.
3. Exogenous infections are caused by PPM introduced to the patient from the environment from either animate or inanimate sources. Following multiplication outside the patient, the PPM are transferred (omitting the first stage of carriage) to the organ where colonisation and infection then occur, e.g. *Pseudomonas* pneumonia following bronchoscopy.

Supercarriage-Colonisation-Infection

Supercarriage-colonisation-infection are the three stages of endogenous infections with a resistant PPM which develops during and after antimicrobial administration.

Clinical Resistance

Clinical resistance is the abnormal carriage of a resistant micro-organism by a patient. This occurs when (a) the antimicrobial minimal inhibitory concentration (MIC) for the colonising or infecting micro-organism is higher than the non-toxic blood concentration after systemic administration or (b) the antimicrobial miniman bactericidal concentration (MBC) for PPM carried in the oropharynx, stomach and gut is higher than the non-toxic concentration achieved after topical administration.

Selective Decontamination of the Digestive Tract

This is a strategy with the aim to eradicate oropharyngeal and gastro-intestinal carriage of PPM by means of lethal salivary and faecal antimicrobial concentrations alone. SDD is only successful if surveillance cultures show that AGNB, yeasts and *S. aureus* are effectively eradicated from the throat, stomach and gut.

Surveillance Samples

Samples from throat and rectum are obtained on admission and afterwards (at least) twice a week. These specimens are needed to detect carriage. This information is crucial for three reasons: (1) to distuinguish exogenous from primary and secondary endogenous infections, (2) to detect abnormal carriage or resistant strains at an "early" stage and (3) to evaluate the efficacy of SDD.

Improving the Outcome of Hospital- and Community-Acquired Pneumonia during Mechanical Ventilation

Eradication of microbes causing organ site infection (i.e. pneumonia) by systemic antibiotics alone is difficult and may even be impossible if the source (oropharynx) of these microbes is not eliminated simultaneously. The impact of SDD on VAP incidence has shown that the source of microbes causing VAP is the oropharyngeal cavity and upper gastro-intestinal tract.

In an integrated approach to the treatment and prevention of infection not only the treatment of local infection with systemic antibiotics is indicated, but also source elimination, i.e. SDD is mandatory.

Critically ill patients in the ICU act as biological amplifiers (oropharingeal and gastro-intestinal carriage preceding organ site colonisation infections) of the microbes present in the environment.

Based on these pathophysiological steps, an integrated approach to pneumonia management in patients on mechanical ventilation consists in the following:

1. *Primary endogenous pneumonia.* Fifty per cent of pneumonias in the ICU are of primary endogenous origin. Micro-organisms already present in the oropharyngeal cavity and upper gastro-intestinal tract of the patient as community-associated bacteria (*H. influenzae, M. catarrhalis, S. aureus, S. pneumoniae*) are the main micro-organisms responsible for CAP. The only way to treat these pneumonias is the timely administration of adequate systemic antibiotics. If patients have been hospitalised in non-ICU wards for lengthy periods in a debilitated condition, the pattern of community-acquired micro-organisms changes and turns into the pattern of hospital micro-organisms, in general AGNB [13]. If pneumonia occurs in such patients, the spectrum of systemic antibiotic treatment should properly cover AGNB. Moreover, treatment of HAP and CAP necessitating ICU treatment with mechanical ventilation should not be complicated by the onset of VAP.

2. *Secondary endogenous pneumonia.* 35 per cent is of secondary endogenous origins. During mechanical ventilation, carriage, colonisation and infection may occur. These types of infection can be prevented by SDD including the oropharyngeal cavity. The efficacy of this manoeuvre in the reduction of secondary

endogenous infections has been shown in two recent meta-analysis studies [8, 9].

3. *Exogenous pneumonia*. 15 per cent VAP is exogenous. Failure of hygienic measures leads to direct inoculation into the bronchial tree of micro-organisms without the preceding step of oropharyngeal carriage [14]. Several potential external sources have been identified: humidifiers, nebulisers, unprotected endobronchial suction, non-sterile instrumentation and the mode of the artificial airway route. This latter point is scientifically neglected. We showed that in patients with a prolonged artifical airway via the orotracheal route under SDD, no colonisation of the bronchial tree occurred, but after changing to the tracheostomy route, colonisation of the lower airways occurred with AGNB in 50% of the patients, while the oropharynx remained effectively decontaminated. This implies an exogeneous development [15]. Improvement of hygienic measures prevented direct exogenous colonisation/infection of the respiratory tract in these patients.

In studies using the SDD approach combined with appropriate systemic antibiotics in established pneumonia on admission (either HAP or CAP), the mortality rates were as low as 12%-15% [16], and these results are strikingly different from the conventional antibiotic treatment strategy.

In CAP needing mechanical ventilation, mortality rates of 22%-33% have recently been reported [16, 17].

The workframe in the ICU at OLVG in patients admitted with pneumonia needing respiratory therapy, including mechanical ventilation and intubation, is a follows:

- Intubation/functional residual capacity (FRC) recruitment.
- Tracheal aspirate for gram stain analysis and culture after intubation.
- Surveillance cultures are obtained to assess the microbiological status of the patient.
- Administration of systemic antibiotics: cefotaxime 4 × 1 g i.v. for CAP and additional tobramycin, quinolones or ceftazidime and metronidazole for HAP; adjustment of antibiotics guided by cultures available on day 2-3 after sampling or based on known epidemiology of resistance patterns in the various hospital wards.
- Initiation of SDD directly after intubation using the PTA (polymyxin, tobramycin, amphotericin) to prevent secondary endogenous pneumonia; on clinical suspicion of opportunistic infections, broncho-alveolar lavage (BAL) diagnostic and empiric antibiotics for *Pneumocystis carini*, *Mycoplasma* or *Legionella*.
- Surveillance cultures of throat/rectum twice a week.
- Cleaning of the artificial airway; renewal of the endotracheal tube in referred patients who have been on mechanical ventilation.
- Nebulisation of antibiotics into the respiratory tract; in the case of AGNB, nebulisation of additional antibiotics (tobramycin 4 × daily 40 mg in 5 ml 0.9 saline, or polymyxin 4 × daily 5 ml = 100 mg) to increase the intrapulmonary concentration of antibiotics.

This protocol based on SDD has been the subject of several meta-analyses indi-

Table 1. Comparison of data from the OLVG and National Database (other ICUs)

	OLVG	Other ICU
Patient with pneumonia (n)	103	229
Age (years)	64.17 ± 16	59.14 ± 18*
APACHE score	19 ± 6.8	20 ± 7 (n.s.)
LOS before ICU (days)	5.3	5.6
LOS in ICU (days)	6.8	12.1**
LOS after ICU (days)	17	15.9
LOS in hospital ICU (%)	28.5	33.6***
Mortality in ICU (%)	14.6	28.4****

Data were collected from 1 January 1998 to 1 July 1999.
APACHE, Acute Physiology and Chronic Health Evaluation; *LOS*, Lenght of stay; *n.s.*, not significant
* $p = 0.01$ (two tailed); ** $p = 0.000$; *** $p = 0.02$; **** $p = 0.008$

cating significant reduction in VAP [odds ratio (OR), 0.35]. A moderate reduction in mortality of 20% was shown [8 ,9].

In patients who already have aerobic gram-negative pneumonia on admission, a high clinical cure rate was obtained with SDD in combination with selected systemic antibiotics [18]. It has been found that CAP or HAP complicated by VAP increases the mortality rate [6].

Data from our unit recently obtained in patients with established pneumonia on admission were compared with outcome data (from the Dutch national database) from other ICU not using this strategy (Tab. 1).

These results indicate that the use of SDD in patients who already have pneumonia on admittance is associated with significantly lower mortality rates than those found in units not using SDD.

Furthermore, these results confirm the observation that VAP in patients with CAP increases mortality [15].

References

1. Heyland DK, Cook DJ, Griffith L et al (1999) The attributable morbidity and mortality of ventilator associated pneumonia in the critically ill patient. Am J Respir Crit Care Med 159:1249-1256
2. Bueno-Cavanillas A, Delgado-Rodrigues M, Lopez-Luque A et al (1994) Influence of nosocomial infections on mortality rate in an intensive care unit. Crit Care Med 22: 55-60
3. Torres A, Aznar R, Gatell JP et al (1990) Incidence risk and prognosis factors of nosocomial pneumonia in mechanically ventilated patients. Am Rev Respir Dis 142:523-528
4. Fagon JY, Chastre J, Vuagnat A et al (1996) Nosocomial pneumonia and mortality among patients in intensive care units. JAMA 275:866-869
5. Fagon JY, Chastre J, Hance AJ et al (1993). Nosocomial pneumonia in ventilated patients: a cohort study evaluating attributable mortality and hospital stay. Am J Med 94:281-288
6. Kollef MH, Silver P, Murphy DM, Trovillion E (1995) The effect of late onset ventilator associated pneumonia in determining patient mortality. Chest 108:1665-1662

7. Rello J, Quintana E, Ausina V et al (1991) Incidence, etiology and outcome of nosocomial pneumonia in mechanically ventilated patients. Chest 100:439-444
8. D'Amico R, Pifferi S, Leonetti C et al (1998) Effectiveness of antibiotic prophylaxis in critically ill adult patients: a systematic review of randomised controlled trials. BMJ 316:1275-1285
9. Nathens AB, Marshall JC (1999) Selective decontamination of the digestive tract in surgical patients: a systematic review of the evidence. Arch Surg 134:170-176.
10. Hammond JMJ, Potgieter PD (1995) Is there a rate for selective decontamination of the digestive tract in primarily infected patients in the ICU? Anaesth Intens Care 23:168-174
11. Leroy O, Guilly J, Georges H et al (1999) Effect of hospital acquired ventilator associated pneumonia on mortality of severe community acquired pneumonia. J Crit Care 13:12-17
12. van Saene HKF, Stoutenbeek CP, Zandstra DF (1992) Eleven important definitions. Rean Urg 1(3 bis):485-487
13. Mobbs KJ, van Saene HKF, Sunderland D et al (1999) Oropharyngeal Gram-negative bacillary carriage in chronic obstructive pulmonary disease: relation to severity of disease. Respir Med 93:540-545
14. Silvestri L, Monti Bragadin C, Milanese M et al (1999) The west ICU. Infection really nosocomial? A prospective observational cohort study of mechanically ventilated patients. J Hosp Infect 42:125-133
15. van der Voort PHJ, Zandstra DF (1996) Kolonisatie van de lage luchtwegen na minitracheostomie tijdens selectieve darmdecontaminatie. Intensive Care Rev 11:213-218
16. Alvarez-Sanchez B, Alvarez Lerma F, Jorda R et al (1998) Prognostic factors and etiology in patients with severe community-acquired pneumonia admitted at the ICU. Spanish multicenter study. Med Clin (Barc) 11(17):650-654
17. Leroy O, Bosquet C, Vandenbussche C et al (1999) Community-acquired pneumonia in the intensive care unit: epidemiological and prognosis data in older people. J Am Geriatr Soc 47(5):539-46
18. Stoutenbeek CP, van Saene HKF, Miranda DR, Zandstra DF (1986) Nosocomial gram-negative pneumonia in critically ill patients. A 3 year experience with a novel therapeutic regimen. Intensive Care Med 12:419

Chapter 2

Diagnostic Tools for Ventilator-Associated Pneumonia

T. Bauer, R. Ferrer, A. Torres

Introduction

Nosocomial pneumonia and ventilator-associated pneumonia (VAP, nosocomial pneumonia after 48 h of mechanical ventilation) are currently the second leading cause of nosocomial infections and account for approximately 10% to 15% of all hospital-acquired infections [1-3]. The incidence of nosocomial pneumonia is increased for all patients in intensive care units (ICU), where respiratory infections have been reported to be the most frequent type of nosocomial infections [4]. During the last 10 years, several diagnostic methods have been developed to microbiologically confirm the clinical diagnosis, especially in mechanically ventilated patients [5]. These methods require the use of bacterial quantitative cultures and for each method a specific bacterial threshold is accepted for the confirmation of a pulmonary infection [6]. However, despite the enormous amount of literature regarding this topic, there is still an open debate about the requirement of invasive fiberoptic bronchoscopic techniques [7-10].

Clinical Diagnosis of VAP

Without clinical suspicion of pneumonia, the physician usually does not request a microbiological work-up. The clinical diagnosis is based on the presence of new and persistent pulmonary infiltrates, fever >38.3°C, leukocytosis, and purulent secretions [11]. Although these parameters are fairly straightforward in nonventilated patients, they frequently present false-positive and false-negative results in patients being mechanically ventilated. Andrews and colleagues, using autopsy results as the gold standard, demonstrated that, according to clinical parameters, acute respiratory distress syndrome (ARDS) is misdiagnosed in 29% of patients [12]. Bell and coworkers, studying similar populations, found 10% false-positive and 62% false-negatives rates [13]. Wunderink et al. did not find a single radiographic sign that demonstrated a diagnostic efficiency higher than 68% [14]. In an immediate postmortem study in which we performed histological analysis of multiple pulmonary biopsies, we found that the single best clinical parameter was pulmonary infiltrates [15]. An effort to improve the diagnostic yield of clinical parameters was made by Pugin et al. [16], who designed a score combining clinical, physiological, and microbiological parameters. Major explanations for false-negative results of clinical parameters rely on the quality deficiencies of portable chest X-ray and in the histological pattern of VAP (diffuse bronchopneumonia), which is not easily detected in the initial periods by portable chest X-ray [17]. False-positive results are explained by the frequent presence of other pulmonary lesions, such as alveolar hemorrhage or diffuse alveolar damage [18].

Invasive Microbiological Methods

The introduction of the flexible fiberoptic bronchoscope in the late 1960s resulted in the ability to directly access lower airways. The most commonly used broncho-scopic methods are the protected specimen brush (PSB) and bronchoalveolar lavage (BAL). The PSB involves positioning the bronchoscope next to the orifice of the sampling area and advancing the PSB catheter 3 cm out of the fiberoptic bron-choscope to avoid collection of pooled secretions on the catheter tip. An inner can-nula is protruded to eject a distal carbon wax plug into the airway, and the catheter is advanced to the desired subsegment. If purulent secretions are visualized, the brush is rotated there. This procedure is necessary to avoid contamination of the brush with microorganisms from the upper respiratory tract [19].

A certain number of brushed secretions may be used for Gram's stain [20], but quantitative bacterial cultures are imperative to distinguish colonization from infection. A growth of 10^3 cfu/ml is considered significant and corresponds to an initial concentration of 10^3 to 10^6 bacteria/ml of the retrieved secretions. The choice of a specific segment for sampling does not appear to affect the sensitivity of the PSB method [21]. However, histological studies have demonstrated that VAP is a multifocal process, suggesting that some of the sensitivity problems of the technique could be related to inherent particularities, such as the segmental sam-pling [22]. Secondly, prior antibiotic therapy is another explanation for false-neg-ative results. Montravers and associates have shown [23] that antibiotics can ster-ilize samples collected by PSB after 3 days of treatment. Thirdly, another possible explanation for false-negative results is that they are not really negative but rather borderline results due to the presence of an early stage of infection. At this stage, withholding antibiotics could be deleterious to patient outcome. Dreyfuss and col-leagues [24] followed up borderline cultures (between 10^2 and 10^3 cfu/ml) and observed that some of these cultures later evolved to positive cultures. Overall, the sensitivity of PSB varies among studies, from 33% to more than 95% with a speci-ficity range from 50% to 100%.

BAL is performed by advancing the bronchoscope distally into a subsegmental bronchus (generally a third- or fourth-generation bronchus) until the airway is occluded proximally. The next step is the instillation of 20- to 50-ml aliquots of sterile saline into the lung periphery, followed by gentle aspiration. As yet, there has been no consensus about the total volume to be instilled, but it is believed that at least 100 ml are required to retrieve secretions from the periphery of the subseg-ment [25]. The sampling area is selected based on the location of the infiltrate on chest X-ray or by direct visualization of a subsegment containing purulent secre-tions. Other methods using protected systems have been designed to avoid conta-mination of the retrieved BAL fluid, hence are more expensive [26]. Quantitative bacterial cultures of BAL fluid are imperative to distinguish colonization from infection ($\geq 10^4$ cfu/ml). Sensitivity of BAL ranges from 22% to 100%. An additional factor that can cause this variability is the repeatability of the method [27].

The examination of BAL fluid for intracellular organisms (ICO) is a specific marker of VAP. The method requires a threshold value of infected cells, usually around 5% [28]. Several studies applied the detection of ICO to assess the diagnostic yield. Sensitivity ranged from 37% to 100%, with a specificity of 89% to 100%.

Noninvasive Microbiological Methods

Several studies have demonstrated that *qualitative* cultures obtained by endotracheal aspirates through a naso- or orotracheal tube or tracheostoma are nonspecific [29]. These cultures are rarely negative in patients beins mechanically ventilated with fever and pulmonary infiltrates, which, in turn, may lead to an overdiagnosis of VAP [30, 31]. The use of *quantitative* cultures of endotracheal aspirates may help avoid false-positive results. The sensitivity for detection of VAP ranges between 50% and 70% and the specificity between 70% and 85%, using thresholds between 10^5 and 10^6 cfu/ml. A good correlation has been demonstrated between *quantitative* cultures of invasive diagnostic methods such as PSB or BAL and endotracheal aspirates [32]. It is an advantage that endotracheal aspirates can be obtained without skilled personnel or equipment, but opponents of this technique argue that the results lead to an excess diagnosis of VAP. However, the rate of false-positive results seems to be similar to invasive techniques when the technique is used with quantitative bacterial cultures [33].

As regards PSB, at least four studies have shown that, when used blindly through an endotracheal tube, this method has a similar accuracy to that of bronchoscopy. One of these studies [34] used the Métras catheter for introducing the PSB and obtaining lower respiratory samples. Pham [35] and colleagues reported that the diagnostic value of quantitative cultures blindly aspirated through a plugged telescoping catheter is similar to that obtained using a PSB via fiberoptic bronchoscopy. The method described by these authors is interesting due to its simplicity and low cost. Blind BAL has been advocated in the form of conventional methods [36], protected catheters using mini-BAL procedures [36], Swan-Ganz catheters [37], or, more recently, protected catheters that can be directed to one or the other side of the lung [38]. Overall, these methods also have an accuracy – when protected – comparable to that of the guided methods.

Side effects of blind diagnostic techniques have not been investigated systematically. However, they are probably like those alluded to above, but with the advantage of avoiding those inherent to the use of fiberoptic bronchoscopy. Moreover, these diagnostic methods have not been extensively validated by postmortem lung examination.

Acknowledgements. Dr. Torsten Thomas Bauer was a research fellow from the Medizinische Klinik, Abteilung für Pneumologie, Allergologie und Schlafmedizin,

Bergmannsheil – Universitätsklinik, Bochum, Germany and was supported in 1999 by *IDIBAPS*, Barcelona, Spain.

Dr. Torres was supported in part by the following grants: Commisionat per a Universitats i Recerca de la Generalitat de Catalunya 1997 SGR 00086, FISS 98/0138, SEPAR 1998, Fundació Clínic / CIRIT, and *IDIBAPS*.

References

1. American Thoracic Society (1996) Hospital-acquired pneumonia in adults: diagnosis, assessment, initial therapy, and prevention: a consensus statement. Am J Respir Crit Care Med 153:1711-1725
2. Barsic B, Beus I, Marton E et al (1999) Nosocomial infections in critically ill infectious disease patients: results of a 7-year focal surveillance. Infection 27:16-22
3. Kampf G, Wischnewski N, Schulgen G et al (1999) Prevalence and risk factors for nosocomial lower respiratory tract infections in German hospitals. J Clin Epidemiol 51:495-502
4. Richards MJ, Edwards JR, Culver DH, Gaynes RP (1999) Nosocomial infections in medical intensive care units in the United States. National Nosocomial Infections Surveillance System. Crit Care Med 27:887-892
5. Bowton DL (1999) Nosocomial pneumonia in the ICU-year 2000 and beyond. Chest 115:28s-33s
6. Reimer LG, Carroll KC (1998) Role of the microbiology laboratory in the diagnosis of lower respiratory tract infections. Clin Infect Dis 26:742-748
7. Niederman M, Torres A, Summer W (1994) Invasive diagnostic testing is not needed routinely to manage suspected ventilator-associated pneumonia. Am J Respir Crit Care Med 150:565-569
8. Chastre J, Fagon JY (1994) Invasive diagnostic testing should be routinely used to manage ventilated patients with suspected pneumonia. Am J Respir Crit Care Med 150:570-574
9. Baughman RP, Tapson V, McIvor A (1999) The diagnosis and treatment challenges in nosocomial pneumonia. Diagn Microbiol Infect Dis 33:131-139
10. Bruchhaus JD, McEachern R, Campbell GDJ (1998) Hospital-acquired pneumonia: recent advances in diagnosis, microbiology and treatment. Curr Opin Pulm Med 4:180-184
11. Johanson WG, Pierce AK, Sanford JP, Thomas GD (1972) Nosocomial respiratory infection with Gram-negative bacilli: the significance of colonization of the respiratory tract. Ann Intern Med 77:701-706
12. Andrews CP, Coalson JJ, Smith JD, Johanson WG (1981) Diagnosis of nosocomial bacterial pneumonia in acute, diffuse lung injury. Chest 80:254-258
13. Bell RC, Coalson JJ, Smith JD, Johanson WG (1983) Multiple organ failure and infection in adult respiratory distress syndrome. Ann Intern Med 99:293-298
14. Wunderink RG, Woldenberg LS, Zeiss J et al (1992) The radiologic diagnosis of autopsy-proven ventilator associated-pneumonia. Chest 101:458-463
15. Fàbregas N, Ewig S, Torres A et al (1999) Clinical diagnosis of ventilator associated pneumonia revisited: comparative validation using immediate postmortem lung biopsies. Thorax 54:867-873
16. Pugin J, Auckenthaler R, Mili N et al (1991) Diagnosis of ventilator associated pneumonia by bacteriologic analysis of bronchoscopic and non-bronchoscopic "blind" bronchoalveolar lavage fluid. Am Rev Respir Dis 143:1121-1129

17. Rouby JJ (1996) Histology and microbiology of ventilator-associated pneumonia. Semin Respir Infect 11:54-60
18. Meduri GU, Mauldin GL, Wunderink RG et al (1994) Causes of fever and pulmonary densities in patients with clinical manifestations of ventilator-associated pneumonia. Chest 106:221-235
19. Wimberley L, Falling LJ, Bartlett JG (1979) A fiberoptic bronchoscopy technique to obtain uncontaminated lower airway secretions for bacterial culture. Am Rev Respir Dis 119:337-343
20. Croce MA, Fabian TC, Waddle-Smith L et al (1998) Utility of Gram's stain and efficacy of quantitative cultures for posttraumatic pneumonia: a prospective study. Ann Surg 227:743-751
21. Marquette CH, Herengt F, Saulnier R et al (1993) Protected specimen brush in the assessment of ventilator-associated pneumonia. Selection of a certain lung segment for bronchoscopic sampling is unnecessary. Chest 103:243-247
22. Fàbregas N, Torres A, El-Ebiary M et al (1996) Histopathologic and microbiologic aspects of ventilator-associated pneumonia. Anesthesiology 84:760-771
23. Montravers P, Fagon JY, Chastre J et al (1993) Follow-up protected specimen brushes to assess treatment in nosocomial pneumonia. Am Rev Respir Dis 147:38-44
24. Dreyfuss D, Mier L, Le Bourdelles K et al (1993) Clinical significance of borderline quantitative protected specimen brush specimen culture results. Am Rev Respir Dis 147:946-951
25. Meduri GU, Chastre J (1992) The standardization of bronchoscopic techniques for ventilator-associated pneumonia. Chest 102:557S-564S
26. Meduri GU, Beals DH, Maijub AG, Baselski V (1991) Protected bronchoalveolar lavage: a new bronchoscopic technique to retrieve uncontaminated distal airway secretions. Am Rev Respir Dis 143:855-864
27. Gerbeaux P, Ledoray V, Boussuges A et al (1998) Diagnosis of nosocomial pneumonia in mechanically ventilated patients: repeatability of the bronchoalveolar lavage. Am J Respir Crit Care Med 157:76-80
28. Torres A, El-Ebiary M, Fàbregas N et al (1996) Value of intracellular bacteria detection in the diagnosis of ventilator associated pneumonia. Thorax 51:378-384
29. Meduri GU (1995) Diagnosis and differential diagnosis of ventilator-associated pneumonia. Clin Chest Med 16:61-93
30. Berger R, Arango L (1985) Etiologic diagnosis of bacterial nosocomial pneumonia in seriously ill patients. Crit Care Med 13:833-836
31. Salata RA, Lederman MM, Shales DM et al (1987) Diagnosis of nosocomial pneumonia in intubated, intensive care unit patients. Am Rev Respir Dis 135:426-432
32. El-Ebiary M, Torres A, González J et al (1993) Quantitative cultures of endotracheal aspirates for the diagnosis of ventilator-associated pneumonia. Am J Respir Crit Care Med 147:1552-1557
33. Chastre J, Fagon JY, Trouillet JL (1995) Diagnosis and treatment of nosocomial pneumonia in patients in intensive care units. Clin Infect Dis 21[Suppl 3]:S226-S237
34. Torres A, Puig de la Bellacasa J, Rodriguez RR et al (1988) Diagnostic value of telescoping plugged catheters in mechanically ventilated patients with bacterial pneumonia using the Metras catheter. Am Rev Respir Dis 138:117-120
35. Pham LH, Brun-Buisson C, Legrand P et al (1991) Diagnosis of nosocomial pneumonia in mechanically ventilated patients: comparison of a plugged telescoping catheter with the protected specimen brush. Am Rev Respir Dis 143:1055-1061
36. Rouby JJ, Rossignon MD, Nicolas MH et al (1989) A prospective study of protected bronchoalveolar lavage in the diagnosis of nosocomial pneumonia. Anesthesiology 71:179-185

37. Gaussorgues P, Piperno D, Bachmann P et al (1989) Comparison of nonbronchoscopic bronchoalveolar lavage to open lung biopsy for the bacteriologic diagnosis of pulmonary infections in mechanically ventilated patients. Intensive Care Med 15:94-98
38. Kollef MH, Bock KR, Richards RD, Hearns ML (1995) The safety and diagnosis accuracy of minibronchoalveolar lavage in patients with suspected ventilator associated pneumonia. Ann Intern Med 122:743-748

Chapter 3

Cost-Effectiveness of New Technology to Reduce Catheter-Related Bloodstream Infections due to Central Venous Catheters

A. SITGES-SERRA

Prevention of Catheter-Related Bloodstream Infections: an Evolving Scenario

Catheter-related bloodsream infections (CRBI) are preventable nosocomial infections. Maximal aseptic barriers at insertion and appropriate site and junction care can reduce this complication to close to zero figures [1-3]. Strict asepsis during catheter manipulation, however, is difficult to implement. Repeated hand washing, the use of sterile gloves during hub handling and appropriate help during nursing are either cumbersome or very expensive for routine use in most centers. Changing personnels shifts, shortage of well-trained health care workers, and low training standards may complicate the situation in many institutions and make effective prevention of CRBI a nightmare. Thus, new prevention strategies are currently being proposed by researchers and manufacturing companies based on "contamination-resistant" devices. The use of these devices is not meant to replace the time-honored principles of prevention based on strict asepsis being implemented at all times; however, new technology may certainly help the health care professionals in reducing sepsis rates. The purpose of this article is to briefly discuss the efficacy of three devices marketed in recent years with the aim of reducing CRBI rates and to presenta data concerning their cost-effectiveness.

Efficacy of New Devices: Impregnated Catheters and Antiseptic Hubs

Antiseptic-Coated Catheters

In 1991, Kamal et al. [4] published a first trial comparing a catheter impregnated with cephazolin with a standard one. Bonding with cephazolin was obtained by pre-treating a conventional catheter with a cationic surfactant. There were no differences in CRBI rates. The prevalence of colonization, however, was significantly reduced (2% vs. 14%). This method did not become popular due to the cumbersome bonding maneuvers and the short duration of the protective effect. The idea, however, was good and shortly afterwards, catheters were manufactured with an external coating of chlorhexidine and silver sulfadiazine (CHX, Arrowguard, Arrow International). These have been tested in several randomized trials with controversial and often negative results [5-11] attributed either to the sterilization process [10] or to the loss of the antiseptic coating [6]. A recent meta-analysis [11] of 12 randomized studies (11 of which failed to show a statistical difference) suggests, however, that CHX may be effective in reducing the CRBI rates (Odds ratio 0.56; $p = 0.005$). In the base-case analysis, use of antiseptic impregnated catheters resulted in a decrease in the incidence of CRBI of 2.2% (5.2% for standard vs. 3.0% for CHX). Accordingly, for future analysis in the present paper, the figure of 40% reduction of CRBI rates will be used to calculate the cost-effectiveness of CHX implementation. A cost-effectiveness analysis of CHX has been recently published [12], suggesting savings ranging from $ 68 to $ 391 per catheter used.

Antibiotic-Coated Catheters

Raad et al. [13] published an initial randomized and double-blind trial of catheters coated with minocycline and rifampin (RM; Cook Spectrum, Cook Critical Care, Bloomington) with a mean indwelling time of 6 days. The incidence of CRBI was significantly reduced from 5% to 0% and that of colonization from 26% to 8%. Later on, the same group [14] conducted a clinical trial comparing CHX with RM with a mean indwelling time of 8 days. The rate of CRBI was significantly lower for RM (0.3% vs. 3.4%; $p < 0.002$). The authors claim that the reason why, in their hands, CHX performed worse than in a previous trial by Maki et al. [9] was mostly due to their using a sonication culture method instead of the semiquantitative rolling method. Sonication recovers microorganisms from both catheter surfaces and thus increases the sensitivity for the diagnosis of CRBI. In addition, it was claimed that the superiority of RM over CHX was also due to the fact that RM are coated on both surfaces while CHX are coated only externally. This would not prevent hub-related endoluminal contamination and increasingly recognized route of catheter contamination [15-17].

Some issues in the Draouiche et al. [14] paper, however, cannot be fully understood. Despite the better protection offered by the RM catheters, the percentage of devices that were withdrawn on the basis of suspicion of CRBI was the same in both groups. There was a rather high rate (15%) of catheters withdrawn for unknown reasons. Finally, a paradoxical result of this study is that, although the mean catheterization time in both groups was 8 days, the actuarial curves of catheters free of CRBI started to diverge from day 10, when only 90 devices per group remained in the study. This suggests that the advantage of RM over CHX is restricted to catheters with indwelling times of over 10 days, when the endoluminal contamination route becomes predominant [16, 18].

RM catheters have not been widely evaluated. Thus, for the purpose of the present study it will be assumed that they will perform 50% as well as they did in the trial [19]. Thus, to simplify matters and for easy calculation purposes, the figure of 90% reduction of CRBI rates will be used to calculate the cost-effectiveness of RM implementation.

Antiseptic Hubs

Strict aseptic manipulation of conventional Luer connectors is cumbersome and expensive. For this reason, protocol violations during catheter manipulations are common. For patients receiving i.v. therapy at home, training becomes painstaking and lack of compliance results in recurrent catheter infections. A current approach to solve the problem of endoluminal contamination is based upon the design of hubs incorporating antibacterial barriers.

A new hub model adopting the piggyback concept and incorporating an antiseptic barrier (3% iodinated alcohol) was developed in our Department of Surgery (SL, Segur-Lock, INIBSA, Barcelona, Spain). In vitro and in vivo studies [20, 21] have shown that purposeful contamination of the male component of the new hub does not result in endoluminal contamination. In a clinical trial, 151 patients with central venous catheterization for a mean of 2 weeks were randomized to receive catheters with standard Luer-lock connectors or protected with SL [22]. CRBI rate was higher in the control group (16% vs. 4%), and this was due to the low rate of hub-related CRBI observed in the group fitted with the new hub (1% vs. 11%, $p <$ 0.01). Handling of junctions equipped with this hub is simplified since it does not require strict asepsis, resulting in substantial savings of dressing time and disposable materials. Other trials evaluating SL are currently in progress.

For calculation purposes, the figure of 75% reduction of CRBI rates, obtained in the only trial conducted on SL, will be used to calculate the cost-effectiveness of SL implementation.

Efficacy of New Devices Depends on Indwelling Time and the Route of Catheter Contamination

CHX catheters are only coated on their external surface. This means that efficacy will be essentially limited against microorganisms present at the skin site and migrating along the external catheter surface. Extraluminal infections occur mostly during the first week of catheterization. Thus, it is not surprising that the published trials show a trend towards benefit for short-term catheterization times [11]. In RM catheters, antibiotics are imbedded in the material and coat both the internal and external surfaces. They may have an advantage in preventing endoluminal contamination, which is particularly relevant after the initial week of catheterization. SL only affords protection against endoluminal contamination and, accordingly, becomes particularly useful after the initial week of treatment.

Cost of the New Devices

The prices of CHX and RM trilumen catheters are currently $ 61 and $ 70 respectively, according to figures published by Darouiche et al. [14]. For the purpose of the present study, a single catheter per patient is evaluated. Scheduled replacement will not be considered.

The price of a Segur-Lock kit (needle and connector) is $ 8. The number of anti-septic connectors used during a single catheterization period depends on the indwelling time and number of times it is accessed. In the present study, a 2-week course treatment with use of only one connector for each lumen of a first genera-tion catheter and a mean of 12 needles a week (for access or during tubing replace-ment) is considered, for a total cost of $ 30 ($ 24 for the antiseptic connectors and $ 6 for needles).

We assume that the cost of a first-generation catheter is $ 20 [19]. Accordingly, the extra cost for prevention per patient is as follows: for CHX $ 41, for RM $ 50 and for SL $ 30.

The Cost of Catheter-Related Bloodstream Infections

This will be calculated on the basis of the papers by Arnow et al. [23] and Morís de la Tassa et al. [24], the first reporting the experience of a North American 450-bed, tertiary center and the second that of a 450-bed European hospital.

Arnow et al. [23] investigated all the episodes of CRBI occurring at the University Chicago Hospital for 4 years. The medical records of the patients were reviewed and the hospital cost for extra medical care related to CRBI calculated and adjusted for inflation to 1991 dollars. During the study period 102 episodes of CRBI were identified. One third of the episodes were caused by coagulase-negative staphylococci, one third by *S. aureus* and, and one third by *Candida* spp. and enteric organisms. One third of the patients sustained a major complication such as septic shock, thrombophlebitis, or metastatic infection. The hospital cost of CRBI averaged $ 3707 per episode in dollars in 1991: $ 1299 for laboratory tests; $ 1437 for therapy and $ 971 for hospital rooms. The average cost for CRBI due to a central venous catheter was $ 2670, which was lower than that for CRBI due to peripheral catheters ($ 4830) and arterial catheters ($ 4464). The hospital cost for CRBI, due to *S. aureus* was $ 6064 and exceeded that for episodes caused by any other pathogens. There were nine episodes of CRBI for which the hospital cost exceeded $ 10000.

For purposes of the present study, based on Arnow's et al. report [23], we have calculated the cost of a CRBI due to a central venous catheter assuming a mean cost of $ 2670 for non-*S. aureus* CRBI and a mean cost of $ 6064 for *S. aureus*-related CRBI. We have also assumed a case mix of two thirds of CRBI due to non-*S. aureus* microorganisms. Finally, we assumed that a 10% increase of costs was indicated to update the 1991 figures to 1999 dollars, compensating for the inflation. Thus, the 1999 mean hospital cost for an episode of central venous CRBI, based on this USA report, has been established to be $ 3850.

Morís de la Tassa et al. [24] conducted a nested case-control study during the years 1993 and 1994. Twenty-two patients with proven CRBI were compared with controls matched for age, sex, fundamental illness, surgical intervention, type of catheter inserted, associated diseases, and date of admission (± 6 months). Half of the CRBI were due to *S. aureus*. As in the study of Arnow et al. [23], costs were assessed for diagnostic tests, therapy, and hospital stay. Hospital stay was almost

Table 1. Resource consumption by patients with catheter-related bloodstream infection compared with matched controls (From [24])

Resource	Cases	Controls	*p*Value
Blood cultures	4.4 ± 2.2	0.25 ± 0.9	0.0001
Urine cultures	1 ± 1	0.3 ± 0.6	0.02
Catheter cultures	0.5 ± 0.6	0.1 ± 0.3	0.01
Blood count	7.7 ± 3.8	4.8 ± 3.7	0.0002
Coagulation tests	1.8 ± 2.1	1.3 ± 1.2	NS
Biochemical tests	5.1 ± 3	4.1 ± 3.3	NS
Fluid therapy (l)	9.4 ± 7.2	4.5 ± 3.5	0.003
Doses of antibiotics	765	150	

NS, not significant

double in patients suffering an episode of CRBI (26 vs. 14 days; $p = 0.0002$). Resource consumption is shown in Table 1. The mean cost of a CRBI episode was established at 536.736 Spanish pesetas, corresponding approximately to $ 3578 in 1995. Increasing this by 8% to compensate for inflation in Spain during the last 3 years, the final figure would be $ 3864. This compares amazingly well with data coming from the USA. Thus, for the purpose of the calculations that will follow on the cost-effectiveness of new catheter technologies, the cost of a "standard episode of CRBI" with a "standard case-mix of microorganisms" will be considered to be $ 3850.

The Cost-Effectiveness of New Catheter Technologies

Tables 2, 3 and 4 show the costs and potential savings due to the implementation of new technologies. They have been drawn on the following basic assumptions:
1. Three baseline or control sepsis rates are exemplified: 2%, 4% and 8%. Overall, the higher the basal sepsis rates are, the higher are also the potential savings.
2. CRBI reduction rates will be considered as follows: 40% for CHX, 90% for RM, and 75% for SL.
3. Extra costs for implementation of new technologies for CRBI prevention have been calculated on the basis of 100 patients and are as follows: $ 4100 for CHX; $ 5000 for RM and $ 3000 for SL.
4. Savings have been calculated as follows:
   Savings = Cost of CRBI in the control group - (Cost CRBI in prevention group + cost of prevention). Thus, a negative result means that overall expenses were higher in the prevention group and, thus, that the implemented device was not cost-effective, while positive figures mean an overall benefit from implementing a particular device.
5. For estimation of the deaths potentially avoided, a 25% attributable death rate will be considered [19].

Table 2. Cost-effectiveness of the implemenation of chlorhexidine-coated catheters (CHX) to prevent catheter-related bloodstream infections (CBRI) in 100 patients

CRBI rates Basal vs. CHX	Prevention cost ($)	Cost CBRI ($) Basal vs. CHX	Savings ($)	Deaths /1000 patients
2% vs. 1.2%	4,100	7,700 vs. 4,620	– 1,020	5 vs. 3
4% vs. 2.4%	4,100	15,400 vs. 9,240	+ 2,060	10 vs. 6
8% vs. 4.8%	4,100	30,800 vs.18,480	+ 8,220	20 vs.12

CHX, chlorhexidine-coated catheters

Table 3. Cost-effectiveness of the implementation of antibiotic-coated catheters (RM) to prevent catheter-related bloodstream infections (CRBI) in 100 patients

CRBI rates Basal vs. CHX	Prevention cost ($)	Cost CBRI ($) Basal vs. CHX	Savings ($)	Deaths /1000 patients
2% vs. 0.3%	5,000	7,700 vs. 1,155	+ 780	5 vs. 0.75
4% vs. 0.6%	5,000	15,400 vs. 2,310	+ 8,090	10 vs. 1.5
8% vs. 1%	5,000	30,800 vs. 3,850	+ 21,950	20 vs. 2.5

CHX, chlorhexidine-coated catheters

Table 4. Cost-effectiveness of the implementation of Segur-Lock (SL) to prevent catheter-related bloodstream infection (CRBI) in 100 patients

CRBI rates Basal vs. CHX	Prevention cost ($)	Cost CBRI ($) Basal vs. CHX	Savings ($)	Deaths /1000 patients
2% vs. 0.5%	3,000	7,700 vs. 1,925	+ 780	5 vs. 1.25
4% vs. 1%	3,000	15,400 vs. 3,850	+ 8,850	10 vs. 2.5
8% vs. 2%	3,000	30,800 vs. 7,700	+ 20,100	20 vs. 5

CHX, chlorhexidine-coated catheters

Conclusions

It is still too soon for a definitive statement concerning the cost-effectiveness of the new devices on the market to reduce the CRBI rates. It seems clear, however, that there are enough data to suggest that these devices will find a definite place in future prevention strategies. More data are needed concerning the efficacy of these devices according to indwelling time and route of catheter contamination. Researchers with no conflicts of interests should independently assess these devices in order to minimize bias due to potential profits from patent holders and manufacturing companies. We urge researchers to implement hub cultures in catheter studies to ascertain the route of catheter contamination, making it possible to assess the efficacy of the devices currently available and others that will surely appear on the market in the near future in relationship to the pathogenesis of CRBI.

It is essential that these new devices be used as a complement and not as a replacement of sterile catheter insertion or manipulation. Furthermore, although the emergence of CRBI due to microorganisms resistant to the antiseptics or antibiotics employed, has, so far, not been a problem, it is essential that the implementation of these devices be appropriately monitored for unusual or unusually resistant pathogens.

Conflict of Interest. Segur-Lock is patent property of the Institut Municipal d'Assistència Sanitària (IMAS), Marcel Segura and Antonio Sitges-Serra. Drs. M. Segura and A. Sitges-Serra are coinventors of Segur-Lock and employed as surgeons by the IMAS. The patent has been licensed to INIBSA, Barcelona, Spain. The IMAS and the inventors receive a percentage of the royalties according to the IMAS official policy but have no other financial links to INIBSA.

References

1. Raad II, Hohn DC, Gilbreath J et al (1994) Prevention of central venous catheter-related infections by using maximal sterile barrier precautions during insertion. Inf Control Hosp Epidemiol 15:231-238
2. Shields PL, Field J, Rawlings J et al (1996) Long-term outcome and cost-effectiveness of parenteral nutrition for acute gastrointestinal failure. Clini Nutri 15:64-68
3. Sitges-Serra A, Pi-Suñer T, Garcés JM, Segura M (1995) Pathogenesis and prevention of catheter-related septicemia. Am J Inf Control 23:310-316
4. Kamal GD, Pfaller MA, Rempe LE, Jebson PJ (1991) Reduced intravascular catheter infection by antibiotic bonding. A prospective, randomized, controlled trial. JAMA 265:2364-2368
5. Pemberton LB, Ross V, Cuddy P et al (1996) No differences in catheter sepsis between standard and antiseptic central venous catheters. A prospective randomized trial. Arch Surg 131:986-998
6. Heard SO, Wagle M, Vijayakumar E et al (1998) Influence of triple-lumen central venous catheter coated with chlorhexidine and silver sulfadiazine on the incidence of catheter-related bacteremia. Arch Int Med 158:81-87
7. Tenneberg S, Lieser M, McCurdy B et al (1997) A prospective randomized trial of an antibiotic and antiseptic-coated central venous catheter in the prevention of catheter related infections. Arch Surg 132:1348-1351
8. Ciresi DL, Albrecht RM, Volkers PA, Scholten DJ (1996) Failure of antiseptic bonding to prevent central venous catheter-related infection and sepsis. Am Surg 62:641-646
9. Maki DG, Stolz SM, Wheeler S, Mermel LA (1997) Prevention of central venous catheter-related bloodstream infection by use of an antiseptic-impregnated catheter. Ann Int Med 127:257-266
10. Sherertz RJ, Heard SO, Raad II et al (1996) Gamma radiation-sterilized, triple lumen catheters coated with a low concentration of clorhexidine were not efficacious at preventing catheter infections in intensive care unit patients. Antimicrob Agents Chemother 40:1995-1997
11. Veenstra DL, Saint S, Lumley T, Sullivan SD (1999) Efficacy of antiseptic-impregnated central venous catheters in preventing catheter-related bloodstream infection: a meta-analysis. JAMA 281:261-267
12. Veenstra DL, Saint S, Sullivan SD (1999) Cost-effectiveness of antiseptic impregnated central venous catheters for the prevention of catheter-related bloodstream infections. JAMA 282:554-560
13. Raad I, Darouiche R, Dupuis J et al (1997) Central venous catheters coated with minocy-

cline and rifampin for the prevention of catheter-related colonization and bloodstream infections. A randomized, double-blind trial. Ann Int Med 127:267-274

14. Darouiche RO, Raad II, Heard SO et al (1999) A comparison of two antimicrobial-impregnated central venous catheters. N Engl J Med 340:1-8
15. Sitges-Serra A, Liñares J, Garau J (1985) Catheter sepsis: the clue is the hub. Surgery 97:355-357
16. Sitges-Serra A, Hernández R, Maestro S et al (1997) Prevention of catheter sepsis: the hub. Nutrition 13:30S-35S
17. Sherertz RJ, Heard SO, Raad II (1997) Diagnosis of triple-lumen catheter infection: comparison of roll plate, sonication, and flushing methodologies. J Clin Microbiol 35:641-646
18. Raad I, Costerton JW, Sabharwall U et al (1993) Ultrastructural analysis of indwelling vascular catheters: a quantitative relationship between luminal colonization and duration of placement. J Inf Dis 168:400-407
19. Wenzel RP, Edmond MB (1999) Editorial. N Engl J Med 340:48-50
20. Segura M, Alía C, Oms L et al (1989) In vitro bacteriological study of a new hub model for intravascular catheters and infusion equipment. J Clin Microbiol 27:2656-2659
21. Segura M, Alía C, Oms L et al (1990) Assessment of a new hub design and the semi-quantitative catheter culture method using an in vivo experimental model of catheter sepsis. J Clin Microbiol 28:2551-2554
22. Segura M, Alvarez F, Tellado JM et al (1996) A clinical trial on the prevention of catheter-related sepsis using a new hub model. Ann Surg 223:363-369
23. Arnow PM, Quimosing EM, Beach M (1993) Consequences of intravascular catheter sepsis. Clin Inf Dis 16:778-784
24. Morís de la Tassa J, Fernández-Muñoz P, Antuña A et al (1998) Estudio de los costes asociados a la bacteriemia relacionada con el catéter. Rev Clin Esp 198:641-646

Chapter 4

Peritonitis: Priorities and Management Strategies

G. Sganga, G. Brisinda, M. Castagneto

Introduction

Despite advances in antimicrobial and surgical therapies, severe peritonitis remains a potentially fatal disease. Furthermore, infections due to spontaneous gastrointestinal perforation and those resulting from injuries or complications of abdominal operations, still represent a challenge for surgeons.

Although a greater understanding of the pathophysiology of intra-abdominal infections, the improvement in critical care and introduction of timed radiological and/or surgical intervention have reduced the mortality associated with severe peritonitis, the rate remains unacceptably high, ranging from 20% to 80% [1-3].

New operative techniques, such as planned relaparotomies, laparostomies or open packing, have introduced an effort to improve the results of treatment of severe intra-abdominal infections, especially those resulting from perforation or anastomotic leakage of the gastrointestinal tract and from infected pancreatitis.

The purpose of this review is to present the state of the art in the management of severe peritonitis, to emphasize persisting controversies, and to identify the gaps in our knowledge that require further study.

Classification and Stratification

Definition

Intra-abdominal infection is defined as an inflammatory response of the peritoneum to micro-organisms and their toxins, which results in purulent exudate in the abdominal cavity. They have two major manifestations: generalized peritonitis and intra-abdominal abscess, a late and localized stage [1-4]. Moreover, peritonitis and intra-abdominal infection are not synonymous.

Intra-abdominal abscess is an intra-abdominal infection that has been confined within the abdominal cavity. Conditions without such peritoneal inflammatory response, in which contamination has occurred but infection is not established (e.g., early bowel perforation), or in which the infectious process remains contained within a diseased, but resectable, organ – such as appendix or gallbladder – represent simple forms of peritonitis, easily cured by an operation and not requiring prolonged additional antibiotic therapy.

Classification

Many attempts have been made to classify peritonitis in general, and secondary peritonitis in particular, which include a large variety of different pathologic conditions, ranging in severity from a local problem to a devastating disease [1, 5-8]. A simplified version of such a classification is presented in Tab. 1. It differentiates between the relatively rare forms of primary peritonitis, which usually respond to medical treatment, and tertiary peritonitis, which does not respond to any treatment, from the commonly occurring secondary peritonitis that mandates surgical intervention [1, 9, 10].

When timely surgical therapy combined with appropriate antimicrobial treatment is undertaken, the infection is resolved in most patients. However, when patients are unable to fight the peritoneal infection, for example, because of an overwhelming infection and impaired defense mechanisms, a diffuse and persistent form of peritonitis – so called tertiary peritonitis – that is often fatal develops. If the infection becomes localized, an intra-abdominal abscess develops [9].

Scoring

The multifaceted nature of severe abdominal infections makes it difficult to precisely define the disease and to assess its severity and to evaluate and compare

Table 1. Classification of intra-abdominal infections

Primary peritonitis
Diffuse bacterial peritonitis in the absence of disruption of gastrointestinal tract
1. Spontaneous peritonitis in children
2. Spontaneous peritonitis in adults
3. Peritonitis in patients receiving continued outpatient peritoneal dialysis
4. Tuberculous and other granulomatous peritonitis

Secondary peritonitis
Localized or diffuse peritonitis originating from a defect in abdominal viscus
1. Acute perforation peritonitis
   A. Gastrointestinal perforation
   B. Intestinal ischemia
   C. Pelviperitonitis and other forms
2. Postoperative peritonitis
   A. Anastomotic leak
   B. Accidental perforation and devascularization
3. Post-traumatic peritonitis
   A. After blunt abdominal trauma
   B. After penetrating abdominal trauma

Tertiary peritonitis
Late peritonitis-like syndrome due to disturbance in the immune response of the patient
1. Peritonitis without evidence of pathogens
2. Peritonitis with fungi
3. Peritonitis with low-grade pathogenic bacteria

therapeutic progress. Both the anatomic source of infection, and to a greater degree, the physiologic compromise it inflicts affect the outcome of the intra-abdominal infection [9-11]. A classification system which accounts for both the anatomical source of the peritoneal infection and the physiological compromise according to the acute physiological score, a part of the Acute Physiology And Chronic Health Evaluation II (APACHE-II) scoring system, has been proposed [12].

The mortality of intra-abdominal infection is related mainly to the severity of the patient's systemic response and the premorbid physiological reserves [7,8,13]. APACHE-II score, which measures the severity of disease, age and chronic health status of the patient, has been validated prospectively in a large number of patients and has been considered as the best available method of risk stratification. However, examining this stratification system, it has been noted that the acute physiological score, malnutrition, and age were noteworthy for predicting outcome, whereas etiology of infection contributed only slightly. Furthermore, the APACHE-II score was independently associated with the mortality rate: patients treated for abdominal infection with a score up to 20 had a risk of death of about 50%.

Microbiology of Peritonitis

Primary peritonitis is a monomicrobial, aerobic infection. It classically occurs in young girls and is caused by *Streptococcus pneumoniae*. In adult patients, the underlying risk factor most frequently encountered is the presence of cirrhosis and ascites. In most cirrhotic patients, bacteriological cultures show *Escherichia coli*. Anaerobes are rare: the presence of obligate anaerobes, or a mixed flora, suggests secondary peritonitis. The latter represents a polymicrobial infection after a spontaneous or traumatic breach in a viscus containing micro-organisms, or because of a postoperative breakdown of intestinal anastomosis. In secondary peritonitis, the infection is most commonly polymicrobial with an average of four isolates per patient, with the most frequently encountered combination being *Escherichia coli* and *Bacteroides fragilis*. The number and types of bacteria increase progressively down the gastrointestinal tract. Proximally, it contains a sparse aerobe (coliforms) and oral anaerobe flora, with the stomach and duodenum normally sterile. However, diseases of the stomach – such as carcinoma, gastric outlet obstruction – or acid-reducing drugs may result in its colonization [14]. Distally, the colon contains the largest concentration of bacteria: after a colonic perforation, more than 400 different species of bacteria invade the peritoneal cavity, although only a few are involved in the ensuing infection [15].

Experimental studies have clarified the pathophysiological mechanisms and the bacteriology of peritonitis, emphasizing the key process of bacterial simplification and synergism [16]. From the initial plethora of contaminating bacteria, the inoculum is spontaneously reduced to include only a few organisms that survive well outside their natural environment: endotoxin-generating facultative anaerobes such as *Escherichia coli*, responsible for the acute peritonitis phase with positive blood cultures, and obligate anaerobes, such as *Bacteroides fragilis*, responsible for late abscess formation. These bacteria act in synergy: both are necessary to produce an abscess, and the obligate anaerobe can increase the lethality of an otherwise nonlethal inoculum of the facultative micro-organism [17, 18]. Consequently, commencing both antiaerobic and antianaerobic treatment reduced the early mortality rate as well as abscess formation. Therefore, in human disease both these agents should be used from the beginning of secondary peritonitis [10].

Postoperative state, administration of systemic and luminal antibiotics, and the invasive environment of the intensive care unit may drastically modify the patient's system, resulting in colonization of the proximal gastrointestinal tract with peculiar micro-organisms (fungi, coagulase-negative staphylococci, and gram-negative bacteria of low pathogenicity). These are the organisms that may be found in tertiary peritonitis, in intensive care unit infections, and in multiple-organ failure [1,9,10,19].

Inflammatory Response in Peritonitis

The outcome of peritonitis depends on the results of a struggle between the systemic and peritoneal defenses of the patient, on one hand, and the nature, volume, and duration of bacterial contamination on the other. The exact events that follow the invasion of the peritoneal cavity with bacteria and adjuvants of infection, such as blood, bile, barium sulfate, and, subsequently, its translymphatic spread, have been clearly defined in recent studies [17,18]. The micro-organisms and their products stimulate the host's cellular defenses to activate a myriad of inflammatory mediators that are responsible for the sepsis [1,18].

Recent molecular biological studies have increased our understanding of the cytokine-mediated inflammatory response in peritonitis. During peritonitis, cytokines (tumor necrosis factor, interleukin-1, interleukin-6, elastase, and others) are measurable in the systemic circulation and in the peritoneal exudates [20,21], and the magnitude of the phenomena is negatively correlated with outcome [21]. Bacterial peritonitis appears to induce an intense compartmentalized inflammatory process. The largest part of peritoneal cytokines probably derive from macrophages exposed to endotoxin liberated from infecting bacteria. Other potential sources are direct translocation of cytokines through the intestinal barrier or production by traumatized tissues [22]. The compartmentalization of the cytokine cascades in peritonitis corroborates the concept that circulating concentrations of cytokines may be misleading and not reflect their tissue concentration or biological activity. Thus, local estimation of cytokines in the peritoneal exudate may better reflect the severity of an initially local process. Timely therapeutic intervention is crucial to abort the ensuing, self-perpetuating systemic inflammatory response syndrome, before overproduction of the mediator nitric oxide completely blocks the Krebs cycle, inflicting advanced injury at the cellular and microvascular level and subsequently leading to multiple organ failure and death [23].

Considerable research effort has been directed, in recent years, at elucidating the role of the gastrointestinal tract and its barrier function in the pathogenesis of severe infections [24]. There is accumulating evidence that sepsis and multiple organ failure in critically ill surgical and injured patients are not always the result of an established infected focus, and that failure of gut barrier function may fuel the systemic component of the systemic inflammatory response syndrome, sepsis, and organ failure. Under these conditions the bacterial translocation, due to gut failure, has been advocated as the trigger of a self-maintaining process for systemic infection and organ failure.

The gut origin hypothesis suggests that a failure of gastrointestinal barrier function, as a results of a major stress insult, permits endotoxin and bacterial translocation through the intestinal wall, which triggers splanchnic cytokines to perpetuate and exacerbate an immunoinflammatory response, first in the immune cells of the intestinal wall, and then in the Kupffer cells and in the reticuloendothelial system. This phenomenon is enhanced by many conditions, and, together with mediator activation and the breakdown of both the macrophage system and the host defense capacity, it results in systemic endotoxemia and/or bacteremia with organ dysfunctions.

Studies in different animal models have shown that bacterial translocation occurs in hemorrhagic shock, thermal injury, malnutrition, endotoxemia, trauma, and intestinal obstruction, and its role in the development of multiple organ failure has been proposed. These studies have demonstrated the presence of bacterial translocation as measured by the recovery of viable enteric organisms from regional lymph nodes, liver, and other organs, increased intestinal permeability to macromolecules, and systemic endotoxemia. In the clinical setting, this hypothesis is still controversial, particularly with respect to bacterial translocation, where there is poor concordance with animal studies. Furthermore, recent papers demonstrate that gut barrier dysfunction occurs after injury, but the magnitude of change does not differentiate patients in whom sepsis develops and those in whom it does not [26]. Other studies failed to demonstrate that gastrointestinal dysfunction is directly linked to sepsis.

Management of Peritonitis

Primary peritonitis is usually treated with antibiotics, not surgically [1, 9, 10]. The goals of the management of secondary peritonitis are summarized in Tab. 2. The three fundamental principles of the surgical management of severe secondary peritonitis are the elimination of the source of the infections, the reduction of bacterial contamination of the peritoneal cavity, and the prevention of persistent or recurrent infections. Nevertheless, intensive measures to support tissue oxygenation and maintain organ function are necessary.

Tertiary peritonitis develops late in the postoperative phase, presents clinically as sepsis, and is associated with a sterile peritoneal cavity or peculiar microbiological findings. Further antimicrobial administration and operative interventions may contribute to the peritoneal superinfection with yeasts and other commensals. The low virulence of these organisms, which represent a marker of tertiary peritonitis and not its cause, reflects the global immunodepression of the affected patients.

Table 2. Principles for the management of peritonitis

Supportive measures
- To combat hypovolemia and shock and maintain adequate tissue oxygenation
- To treat bacteria not eliminated by surgery with antibiotics
- To support failing organ systems
- To provide adequate nutrition

Operative treatment
- Repair and/or control the source of infection
- Evacuate bacterial inoculum, pus, and adjuvants
- Treat abdominal compartment syndrome
- Prevent or treat persistent and recurrent infection or verify both repair and purge

Antibiotic Therapy

Several studies have identified *Escherichia coli* and *Bacteroides fragilis* as the main target organisms for antibiotic therapy. The current practice of early empirical administration of antibiotics targeted against these bacteria is well established [27]. However, issues concerning the choice and timing of drugs, the need for operative cultures, and the duration of postoperative administration are controversial.

Unfortunately, prospective and randomized studies on antibiotic management of peritonitis failed to provide reliable information because the patients whose illnesses are most severe usually are excluded by study design. In many trials, however, low mortality-penetrating trauma cases, that represent contamination rather than infection, have been included. Consequently, the average mortality rate in the antibiotics studies was only 3.5% [28]. This sharply contrasts with the 30% average mortality rate, which is consistently associated with severe infections [1,9,10].

Although several options have been proposed, antibiotic therapy for secondary peritonitis is simple: the emerging concepts suggest that less, in terms of the number of drugs and the duration of treatment, is better. To hit *Escherichia coli*, an antibiotic that kills all strains and, thus does not induce resistance, is required: third-generation cephalosporins such as cefotaxime sodium, ceftizoxime sodium, cefmenoxime hydrochloride, and ceftriaxone sodium meet this requirement.

Recent studies [10, 29] suggest that monotherapy with a single broad-spectrum antibiotic that includes full activity against *Escherichia coli* may be equal or superior to polytherapy with multiple drug combinations. Because monotherapy has not been studied adequately in patients with established peritonitis of intestinal or postoperative origin, and because many of the b-lactam antibiotics are not fully effective against obligate anaerobes in the peritoneal cavity [27], the addition of metronidazole to an antiaerobic agent has been advocated. The active compound of cilastatin-imipenem is an effective sole agent for severe intra-abdominal infection [30]. It should be reserved, however, as a second-line agent for the nosocomially altered spectrum of postoperative peritonitis.

The value of obtaining routine intraoperative peritoneal cultures has become questionable because the results rarely influence clinical decisions, and usually are available only when therapy is no longer necessary. Moreover, the trend to continue administration of antibiotics for fixed periods is no longer justified. The conditions representing simple peritoneal infections (simple cholecystitis, appendicitis) or contamination do not require prolonged postoperative antibiotics. Further changes in current practice are being examined to possibly minimize postoperative administration by intraoperative stratification of the extent of infection, tailoring the duration of therapy to operative findings [31].

Surgical Therapy

The operative approach and the surgical strategy depend on the source of the infection, the degree of peritoneal contamination, the clinical condition of the patient, and the concomitant disease. This approach reduced mortality from 90% to approximately 40% [1,10]. Ideally, a severe intra-abdominal infection should be cured with a single surgical procedure; unfortunately, infection often persist or recurs in cases of severe peritonitis.

Traditionally, severe peritonitis has been approached by performing a midline laparotomy to identify and eliminate the source of infection. Frequently, it involves a simple procedure, such as appendectomy. Occasionally, major resections, such as gastrectomy or colectomy, are indicated. Generally, the choice of the procedure, and whether the ends of resected bowel are anastomosed, exteriorized, or simply closed depends on the anatomic source of infection, the degree of peritoneal inflammation and generalized septic response, and the patient's premorbid reserves. No formula is available, but the prevailing trend has been to minimize the immediate risk of complications by avoiding any intestinal suture lines in the presence of severe peritonitis [1, 9, 10]. In certain instances, such as in severe, infected pancreatic necrosis, complete control of the infective focus is not feasible during the first operation.

The second goal of surgical management of severe peritonitis is the reduction of bacterial contamination. All intraperitoneal fluids should be aspirated, and particulate matter should be removed. Pelvic regions, paracolic gutters and subphrenic spaces must be opened and debrided. Although appealing and popular with surgeons, there is no evidence that intraoperative peritoneal lavage reduces mortality or the incidence of septic complications in patients receiving adequate systemic antibiotics [32]. Peritoneal irrigation with antibiotics is not advantageous because bacteria need to be exposed to the antibiotic for hours to be effective. The addition of antiseptics may even produce toxic effects. Intraperitoneal instillation of heparin has decreased mortality in a few experimental studies; however, no clinical trials are available. In absence of clear benefit, it has been suggested that the lavage fluid is completely aspirated before abdominal closure.

The concept of radical debridement of the peritoneal cavity did not withstand the test of a prospective randomized study because aggressive debridement caused excessive bleeding from the denuded peritoneum and endangered the integrity of the friable intestine. The role of postoperative peritoneal lavage is questionable because the basic question remains of whether it is possible to irrigate the whole abdominal cavity. Drains still are commonly used and misused; they can erode into intestine or blood vessels and promote infective complications [33]. Their use should be limited to the evacuation of an established abscess, to allow the escape of potential visceral, biliary, and pancreatic secretions and to establish a controlled intestinal fistula when the latter cannot be exteriorized [10,33].

Despite gradual improvement in intensive care and antimicrobial therapy, it has become clear that if the initial standard operation fails, persisting or recurrent intra-abdominal infection sometimes may be overlooked or the diagnosis delayed [34]. Waiting for the appearance of signs of persisting infection or organ failure as the indication for abdominal re-exploration *on demand* often proved futile. To improve results, two therapeutic concepts have been introduced: open management, so called laparostomy [35, 36], and planned relaparotomies [37, 38], in which multiple operative interventions are planned before or during the first procedure for peritonitis, to return to the abdominal cavity to re-explore, evacuate, debride, or resect. Reoperations are performed at fixed intervals, irrespective of the clinical condition of the patient, to prevent development of further septic fluid collections, thus precluding systemic effects. Adverse effects of planned relaparotomies are frequent and include damage to abdominal wall structures and intra-peritoneal viscera, causing bleeding or even enteric fistulas.

Open management facilitates frequent re-exploration and, by treating the entire peritoneal cavity as one large infected collection, continuous exposure for maximal drainage. Furthermore, it serves to decompress the high intra-abdominal pressure caused by peritoneal edema associated with inflammation and fluid resuscitation, thus obviating the deleterious systemic consequences of abdominal compartment syndrome [39]. Early results of these methods were promising, particularly in the management of infected pancreatic necrosis, but were less favorable in cases of postoperative peritonitis. Simple open management was plagued by intestinal fistulas and abdominal wall defects [40], problems that were almost eliminated by introduction of temporary abdominal closure devices such as the artificial mesh-zipper techniques. Staged abdominal repair as a conceptual operative approach combines the advantages of planned relaparotomy and of open management with a minimal rate of complications. Prospective, nonrandomized attempts to compare closed and open techniques did not demonstrate an advantage of the latter. Furthermore, recent series failed to to demonstrate the benefits of planned relaparotomies. However, another prospective study showed the staged abdominal repair approach to be superior to conventional operative therapy when patients at equal mortality risk were compared. It has been shown in trauma cases that repeated operations performed in patients in whom the inflammatory response is already active may precipitate multiorgan dysfunction. Besides, these techniques may be beneficial if initiated early, in well-selected patients, for specific indications (Tab. 3), performed by a team of dedicated surgeons.

Management of Intra-Abdominal Abscess

Abscess represents a relatively successful outcome of peritonitis. It may be visceral and nonvisceral, extra- or intra-peritoneal. Nonvisceral abscesses arise after res-

Table 3. Indications for staged abdominal repair

- Critical patient condition (hemodynamic instability) precluding definitive repair
- Excessive peritoneal edema (abdominal compartment syndrome; pulmonary, cardiac, renal, or hepatic dysfunction, and decreased visceral perfusion) preventing abdominal closure without under tension, intra-abdominal pressure > 15 mmHg
- Massive abdominal wall loss
- Impossibility to eliminate or to control the source of infection
- Incomplete debridement of necrotic tissue
- Uncertainty of viability of remaining bowel
- Uncontrolled bleeding (the need for "packing")

olution of diffuse peritonitis in which a loculated area of suppuration persists, or after a perforation of a viscus that is effectively localized by peritoneal defenses. Percutaneous, ultrasound, or computed tomography-guided drainage is the method of choice for single abscesses. Although retrospective studies do not attribute lower mortality or morbidity rates to percutaneous drainage versus surgical drainage [41], the former represents a minimally invasive procedure that can spare the patient the unpleasantness of another open abdominal operation. Furthermore, percutaneous catheter drainage should be considered as the initial therapy for patients with culture-positive peripancreatic fluid collection [42]. Mutiloculated abscesses associated with tissue necrosis, enteric communication, or tumor require laparotomy. Failure of percutaneous drainage indicates that surgery is urgently required.

References

1. Bosscha K, van Vroonhoven JMV, van der Werken C (1999) Surgical management of severe secondary peritonitis. Br J Surg 86:1371-1377
2. Goris RJA, te Boekhorst TPA, Nuytinck JKS, Gimbrere JSF (1985) Multiple-organ failure: generalized autodestructive inflammation? Arch Surg 120:1109-1115
3. Marshall JC, Sweeney D (1990) Microbial infection and the septic response in critical illness. Arch Surg 125:17-23
4. Bone RG, Balk RA, Cerra FB et al (1992) Definitions for sepsis and organ failure and guidelines for the use of innovative therapies in sepsis. The ACCP/SCCM Consensus Conference Committee. American College of Chest Physicins/Society of Critical Care Medicine. Chest 101:1644-1655
5. Wittmann DH, Walker AP, Condon RE (1993) Peritonitis, intra-abdominal infection, and intra-abdominal abscess. In: Schwartz SI, Shires GT, Spencer FC (eds) Principles of surgery, 6th edn. McGraw-Hill, New York, pp 1449-1484
6. Wittmann DH (1990) Symposium of intra-abdominal infections: introduction. World J Surg 14:145-148
7. Rotstein OD, Meakins JL (1990) Diagnostic and therapeutic challenges of intra-abdominal infections. World J Surg 14:159-166
8. Rotstein OD, Simmons RL (1994) Peritonitis and intraabdominal abscess. In Barie PS, Shires GT (Eds) Surgical Intensive Care. Little Brown, Boston, pp 1043-1063

9. Schein M (1992) Management of severe intra-abdominal infection. Surg Annu 24:47-68
10. Wittmann DH, Schein M, Condon RE (1996) Management of secondary peritonitis. Ann Surg 224:10-18
11. Bohnen J, Boulanger M, Meakins JL, McLean AP (1983) Prognosis in generalized peritonitis: relation to cause and risk factors. Arch Surg 118:285-290
12. Meakins JL, Solomkin JS, Allo MD et al (1984) A Proposed classification of intra-abdominal infections. Arch Surg 119:1372-1378
13. Knaus WA, Draper EA, Wagner DP, Zimmerman JE (1985) APACHE II: a severity of disease classification system. Crit Care Med 13:818-829
14. Finegold SM (1982) Microflora of the gastrointestinal tract. In: Wilson SE, Finegold SM, Williams RA (eds) Intra-abdominal infection. McGraw-Hill, New York, pp 1-22
15. Krepel CJ, Gohr CM, Edmiston CE, Condon RE (1995) Surgical sepsis: constancy of antibiotic susceptibility of causative organisms. Surgery 117:505-509
16. Bartlett JG, Onderdonk AB, Louie TJ, Kasper DL (1978) A review: lesson from an animal model of intra-abdominal sepsis. Arch Surg 113:853-857
17. Maddaus MA, Ahrenholz D, Simmons RL (1988) The biology of peritonitis and implications for treatment. Surg Clin North Am 68:431-433
18. Parrillo JE (1993) Pathogenic mechanisms of septic shock. N Engl J Med 328:1471-1477
19. Marshall JC, Christou NV, Meakins JL (1993) The gastrointestinal tract: the "undrained abscess" of multiple organ failure. Ann Surg 218:111-119
20. Holzheimer RG, Schein M, Wittmann DH (1995) Inflammatory mediators in plasma and peritoneal exudate of patients undergoing staged abdominal repair (STAR) for severe peritonitis. Arch Surg 130:1314-1320
21. Gabay C, Kushner I (1999) Acute-phase proteins and other systemic responses to inflammation. N Engl J Med 340:448-454
22. Deitch EA (1993) Cytokines yes, cytokines no, cytokines maybe? Crit Care Med 21:817-819
23. Palmer RMJ (1993) The discovery of nitric oxide in the vessel wall. Arch Surg 128:396-401
24. Sganga G, Gangeri G, Montemagno S, Castagneto M (1994) Prevention of translocation – prevention of multiple organ system failure. In: Mutz NJ, Koller W, Benzer H (eds.) Proceedings of the 7th European Congress on Intensive Care Medicine. Monduzzi, Bologna, pp 93-101
25. Moore FA (2000) Common mucosal immunity: a novel hypothesis. Ann Surg 231:9-10
26. Kanwar S, Windsor ACJW, Welsh F et al (2000) Lack of correlation between failure of gut barrier function and septic complications after major upper gastrointestinal surgery. Ann Surg 231:88-95
27. Wittmann DH, Bergstein JM, Frantzides CT (1991) Calculated empiric antimicrobial therapy for mixed surgical infections. Infection 19 [Suppl 6]:345-350
28. Solomkin JS, Meakins JL, Dellinger EP (1984) Antibiotics trials in intra-abdominal infections: a critical evaluation of study design and outcome reporting. Ann Surg 201:29-39
29. Hopkins JA, Wilson SE, Bobey DG (1994) Adjunctive antimicrobial therapy for complicated appendicitis: bacterial overkill by combination therapy. World J Surg 18:933-938
30. Solomkin JS, Dellinger EP, Christou NV, Busuttil RW (1990) Results of a multicenter trial comparing imipenem/cilastatin to tobramycin/clindamycin for intra-abdominal infections. Ann Surg 212:581-591
31. Schein M, Assalia A, Bachus H (1994) Minimal antibiotic therapy after emergency abdominal surgery: a prospective study. Br J Surg 81:989-891

32. Schein M, Cecelter G, Freinkel W, Gerding H (1990) Peritoneal lavage in abdominal sepsis: a controlled clinical study. Arch Surg 125:1132-1135
33. Farthmann EH, Schöffel U (1990) Principles and limitations of operative management of intraabdominal infections. World J Surg 14:210-217
34. Barendregt W, de Bower H, Kubat K (1992) The results of autopsy of patients with surgical disease of the digestive tract. Surg Gynecol Obstet 175:227-232
35. Steinberg D (1979) On leaving the peritoneal cavity open in acute generalized suppurative peritonitis. Am J Surg 137:216-220
36. Schein M, Saadia R, Decker GG (1986) The open management of the septic abdomen. Surg Gynecol Obstet 163:587-591
37. Penninckx FM, Kerremans RPJ, Lauwers PM (1983) Planned relaparotomies in the surgical treatment of severe generalized peritonitis from intestinal origin. World J Surg 7:762-766
38. Teichmann W, Wittmann DH, Andreone A (1986) Scheduled reoperations (Etappenlavage) for diffuse peritonitis. Arch Surg 121:147-152
39. Schein M, Wittmann DH, Aprahamian C, Condon RE (1995) Abdominal compartment syndrome: the physiological and clinical consequences of elevated intra-abdominal pressure. J Am Coll Surg 180:745-753
40. Kinney EV, Polk HC (1987) Open treatment of peritonitis: an argument against. Adv Surg 21:19-28
41. Levison MA, Zeigler D (1991) Correlation of APACHE II score, drainage technique and outcome in postoperative intra-abdominal abscess. Surg Gynecol Obstet 172:89-94
42. Baril NB, Ralls PW, Wren SM et al (2000) Does an infected peripancreatic fluid collection or abscess mandate operation? Ann Surg 231:361-367

Chapter 5

Bacterial Translocation

G. SGANGA, H.K.F. VAN SAENE, G. BRISINDA, M. CASTAGNETO

Introduction

The pathophysiology of sepsis and multiple organ failure (MOF) remains the subject of intense investigation, and, despite extensive studies, MOF is still a clinical dilemma. The syndrome involves the progressive – and sometimes sequential – dysfunction of physiologic systems in the presence of a clinical picture of systemic sepsis [1-4]. It occurs with distressing frequency in patients after treatment of major injuries and operations for intra-abdominal emergencies or sepsis, and its mortality rate increases progressively with the number of organs involved [2, 3]. Furthermore, the pathophysiology of this syndrome and, thus, specific prophylaxis and treatment remain elusive, and the disappointing results of recent clinical trials of anti-endotoxin antibodies emphasize the incomplete understanding of this problem [5].

Several hypotheses have been set forth to explain a common end-organ injury that results from different etiologies. Moreover, several organs are involved in the pathogenesis of MOF: some are considered to be target organs, damaged by systemic and local inflammatory activation [2, 3], others seem to favor the beginning or the progression of MOF. Such distinction is quite artificial: an organ can initially be the target of damage and then become a motor organ that promotes the persistence of MOF.

Considerable research effort has been directed in recent years at elucidating the role of the gastrointestinal tract (GIT) and its barrier function in the pathogenesis of severe nosocomial infections [6-11]. There is accumulating evidence that sepsis and MOF in critically ill surgical and injured patients are not always the result of an established infected focus, and that a failure of GIT barrier function may fuel the systemic component of the systemic inflammatory response syndrome (SIRS), sepsis, and organ failure. In these conditions the bacterial translocation (BT), due to gut failure, has been advocated as the trigger of a self-maintaining process for systemic infection and MOF [1-3].

The gut origin hypothesis suggests that a failure of GIT barrier function, as a result of a major stress insult, allows endotoxin and BT to penetrate the intestinal wall, which triggers splanchnic cytokines to perpetuate and exacerbate an immunoinflammatory response, first in the immune cells of the intestinal wall, and then in the Kupffer cells and in the reticuloendothelial system. This phenomenon is enhanced by many conditions, which together with the mediator activation and the breakdown of both the macrophage system and the host defense capacity result in systemic endotoxemia and/or bacteremia with organ dysfunction.

Studies in different animal models have shown that BT occurs in hemorrhagic shock, thermal injury, malnutrition, endotoxemia, trauma, intestinal obstruction, and its role in the development of MOF has been proposed [1-4]. These studies have demonstrated the presence of BT as measured by the recovery of viable enteric organisms from regional lymph nodes, liver, and other organs, increased intestinal permeability to macromolecules, and systemic endotoxemia. In the clinical setting this hypothesis is still controversial, particularly with respect to BT, where there is poor concordance with animal studies [2, 3]. Furthermore, recent papers demonstrated that gut barrier dysfunction occurs after injury, but the magnitude of change does not distinguish between patients in whom sepsis develops and those in whom it does not [12]. Other studies failed to demonstrate that GIT dysfunction is directly linked to sepsis. This review summarizes recent data on BT and its role in the onset of MOF. We consider whether prevention of translocation can prevent systemic infection, organ dysfunction, and subsequent mortality related to MOF.

Pathophysiology of MOF

MOF develops mostly in critically ill patients with severe homeostasis disorders, and is characterized by sequential, multiple and progressive impairment in the function of multiple organs and systems. It can follow several injury states, such as hemorrhagic shock, sepsis, large burns, pancreatitis, multiple trauma, respiratory distress syndrome, and complicated surgery [1-3].

In spite of the initial etiologic factor, MOF is considered to start as a consequence of an excessive, uncontrolled, and prolonged activation of the inflammatory system, as a consequence of a generalized autodestructive inflammation [7]. However, MOF appears to be so strongly correlated with sepsis that its development must indicate an occult septic focus.

Sepsis is characterized by an intense activation of several immuno-inflammatory systems, which leads to the release of multiple soluble mediators. This stress-activated biohumoral response plays a major role in the pathophysiologic and metabolic changes, acts as mechanism for host defenses, and promotes tissue repair and recovery from the injury. The released mediators include cytokines (TNF, IL, IFN), complement, oxygen free radicals, proteases, PAF, nitric oxide (NO), and eicosanoids [2, 3].

Recently, NO has emerged as an important mediator of gut failure. In particular, evidence suggests that NO regulates mucosal blood flow, mucosal protection, hemodynamic responses to liver disease, hepatocyte synthetic function, and relaxation of the muscles. NO also regulates agonist-mediated increases in blood flow. Additional results indicate that endogenous NO may interact with prostacyclin and vasodilatory neuropeptides to regulate gastric mucosal integrity. The mechanism underlying the mucosal protective effects of NO is unknown. Current data, however, have been derived entirely from animal models, and as a consequence, the role of NO in human GIT mucosal blood flow is not well defined.

NO has also been implicated in the maintenance of microvascular integrity of the intestinal mucosa after challenge with endotoxin. In the rat, intravenous endotoxin results in acute intestinal vascular damage, vasocongestion, and plasma exudation into the intestinal lumen. Recent evidence suggests that NO may protect against the sequelae of endotoxin-induced shock. It is hypothesized that NO aids in the maintenance of microvascular integrity and flow in the setting of endotoxin administration, although the mechanism remains obscure.

Furthermore, NO can modulate leukocyte-endothelial interactions. Recent data suggest that NO may regulate molecular components of leukocyte sequestration and activation and, as a result, may play a role in ischemia-reperfusion injury and endotoxin-induced shock.

Others have speculated that NO interacts with the superoxide anion to produce a less toxic species. Thus, the mechanism for the mucosal protective effect of NO in endotoxin-induced shock is unknown, but may involve free radical detoxification, leukocyte adhesion properties, and microvascular hemodynamic regulation.

In the setting of MOF, patients often manifest hepatocellular dysfunction, such as elevated bilirubin and decreased serum albumin. Although the mechanism is unclear, it has been suggested that hepatocyte dysfunction is the result of cytokine-induced mediator release by macrophages or Kupffer cells. NO has been targeted as a regulatory mediator.

Leukocytes and macrophages play a central role in the immunobiologic response to injury and infection. They are activated from bacteria, endotoxin, necrotic tissue, ischemia, and other inflammatory stimuli. The activated cellular pool synthesizes and releases the most important humoral mediators and modulates the entire immuno-inflammatory response. An exaggerated and continued stimulation of these cells can produce an uncontrolled endogenous host response, with subsequent, excessive mediator production and autodestructive inflammatory damage at multisystemic levels [13].

The gut has emerged as a central organ in the pathophysiology of MOF. GIT dysfunction may be an effect of shock, but it may also be an important cause of the perpetuation of various shock syndromes. In fact, the former is a potential source of bacteria and toxins, which can spread to the bloodstream as a consequence of anatomical or functional impairment of the intestinal mucosa, producing clinical sepsis without a septic focus, and the latter has a critical function in preserving the patient's defense mechanisms and plays a key role in modulating the inflammatory response [2, 3, 13].

The liver filter can be passed in particular when its function is already impaired by other mechanims, such as hypoperfusion, hypoxia, and primary liver diseases: Kupffer cell failure can result in bacterial killing and clearance deficiency, detrimental mediator effects, and onset of MOF. In this hypothesis the gut acts as the starter and the liver as the motor of MOF [14].

Pathophysiology of Gut Failure and Bacterial Translocation

Several experimental studies show that the small bowel becomes a target after any type of injury, and its dysfuction leads to altered permeability with increased bacterial and endotoxin absorption. By definition, BT is the passage of viable and non-viable bacteria and/or their toxic bioproducts through the intestinal mucosa to the mesenteric lymph nodes, spleen, liver, and peritoneum [2,3,13].

It is currently accepted that indigenous bacteria translocate continuously from the normal GIT, but in low concentration, and the host immune system is able to destroy them prior to systemic spread. This process allows the whole organism to maintain a natural immunity to a variety of pathogens.

In this chapter we consider the hypothesis that BT can be followed by a spreading into the systemic bloodstream, leading to systemic sepsis and MOF.

BT is always related to an interruption of the GIT barrier as a consequence of functional and/or anatomical damage to the intestinal mucosa, the so-called gut failure [2, 3].

The gut barrier has both extrinsic and intrinsic components [1-3, 13]: the extrinsic barrier, located within the lumen, stabilizes the microenvironment at the epithelial surface and consists of mucous, secretory IgA, the unstirred layer, and the luminal flora; the intrinsic components are represented by the epthelial cells and by the spaces around them, which are protected by tight junctions. These components of the GIT barrier can be very easily passed in case of mucosal disruption.

In critically ill patients with severe homeostasis disorders, many different factors are involved in the pathophysiology of bacteria and endotoxin translocation, either in conditions of anatomically intact bowel barrier or in conditions of altered intestinal mucosa (Tab. 1). All these factors provide the intraluminal contents of the intestine with ready access to extraintestinal sites. The exact mechanism of translocation, however, has not yet been completely elucidated.

With regard to the potential involvement of the gut in the pathogenesis of MOF,

Table 1. Factors involved in the pathophysiology of bacterial translocation

Pathophysiological events	Causes
Inadequate oxygen delivery to GIT tissue	Local hypoperfusion Hypodynamic states
Local ischemia Microcirculatory impairment	Bowel distention Vasoconstriction
Mucosal atrophy and overgrowth of GIT flora	Oral feeding discontinuation TPN Protein catabolism Deficiency in glutamine pool
Inflammatory damage and intestinal stasis	Neutrophil activation Oxygen free radical production Mediator release
Decreased host defense mechanism	Immunosoppression Malnutrition

a novel hypothesis has been recently proposed [8]. Shock (via ischemia/reperfusion injury and inhibitory neuroendocrine reflexes) and emergency laparotomy (via anesthesia and bowel manipulation) can cause an early ileus. Disuse (parenteral instead of enteral nutrition) and intensive care unit (ICU) therapies promote further GIT dysfunction, characterized by progressive ileus, colonization of the upper gut, increased permeability, and decreased function of the gut-associated lymphoid tissue. Consequently, the upper GIT becomes a reservoir for pathogens, and local and systemic defense mechanisms that prevent the spread of these organisms are impaired; the primary route of dissemination is not clear.

Alexander and co-workers [15] captured the process of microbial translocation by using an electron and light photomicrography in an excluded loop of terminal ileum from a burned guinea pig after the introduction of *Candida albicans* in its lumen. Therefore, GIT should not be considered as a passive organ [16, 17] but as a dynamic organ whose function covers the traditional role in nutrient absorption together with a front-line defense against the potential detrimental effect of the intestinal flora. Its failure to act as an effective barrier may initiate or exacerbate sepsis in surgical patients [8,18]. Therefore, the maintenance of gut barrier function is recognized as an important goal in the management of high-risk surgical patients [2, 3].

In healthy subjects, the proximal GIT is sterile, or sparsely populated with a relatively avirulent flora. Critical illness is associated with significant proximal gut overgrowth with typical pathogens, and this pathologic colonization contributes significantly to the development of ICU-acquired infection. Furthermore, up to 90% of the patients with ICU-acquired infection had at least one episode of infection with an organism that was simultaneously present in the upper GIT. The hypothesis that GIT carriage sets the stage for the development of invasive infection is supported by two recent meta-analyses of randomized SDD-trials showing a significant reduction in pneumonia and septicemia by 65 and 50%, respectively [19-21].

The relative sterility of the upper GIT is maintained through the interaction of a number of factors (gastric acidity, normal motility, bile salts, IgA, and defensins from Paneth cells). Enteral feeding is a potent stimulus to the activation of normal proximal gut antimicrobial defenses, stimulating gastric acid release, bile flow, and small intestinal motility; cholecystokinin and secretin release, in turn, contributes augmenting mucosal IgA production by the small bowel. Critical illness is associated with profound disruption of these normal defenses. Furthermore, a reduction in rates of nosocomial infection has been observed when enteral nutrition (TEN) is instituted early [10].

The indigenous flora exerts an important influence in rendering the gut resistant to colonization with exogenous pathogens, the so-called colonization resistance. Disruption of the normal flora by antibiotics can reduce colonization resistance and promote pathologic colonization. However, invasive infection with organisms colonizing the upper GIT has been observed. Concomitant colonization of an infected wound and the upper GIT may simply reflect a process of generalized epithelial colonization, unrelated to the development of systemic infection. Some of the cases of tertiary peritonitis may have been secondary to bacterial passage through anatomic defects in the gut, although few patients with this complication demonstrated macroscopic communication between the gut and the peritoneal cavity. The organisms isolated from these cases – coagulase-negative *Staphylococci, Candida, Pseudomonas, Enterococcus* – are typically seen in recurrent, tertiary peritonitis. These organisms have all been shown to be capable of translocation across an anatomically intact GIT in animal models. Moreover, factors known to promote BT (trauma, endotoxemia, parenteral feeding, cholestasis, and use of broad-spectrum antibiotics) are commonly present in critically ill surgical patients [6].

Whether the relationship between GIT colonization and systemic infection reflects cause and effect or simply association, it is apparent that the microbial environment of the critically ill patient is well reflected in the patterns of gut colonization that evolve during the ICU stay. Moreover, the strong correlation between pathologic GIT colonization, ICU-acquired infection, and MOF evolution justifies the conceptual characterization of the GIT as the undrained abscess of MOF [1-3, 11].

The Role of Gut Failure and Bacterial Translocation in the Onset of MOF

GIT has been viewed in the past as a passive organ with just a nutritional function that must be put to rest and can be effectively substituted with total parenteral nutrition (TPN). In the last decade, a considerable body of evidence has been accumulated that GIT plays an important role in the pathophysiology of shock states, and that the damage of intestinal mucosa can result in intraluminal bacteria penetration in the venous and lymphatic vessels. In fact, GIT is responsible for several metabolic and immunobiological functions, and in particular it acts as a barrier against bacteria and their toxins.

There is also accumulating evidence that sepsis and MOF in critically ill surgical and injured patients is not always the result of an established infected focus. In these clinical conditions, the gut failure and the BT have been advocated as the trigger and the self-maintaining process for systemic infection and MOF [2, 3].

In order to establish the dangerous effects of BT, the critical functional activity of the lymphoid tissue in the intestinal wall and in the regional limph nodes, the activation of the Kupffer cells in the liver and the alveolar macrophages in the lungs have been considered. The first step is the activation of immunologic cells of the intestinal wall, followed by the involvement of regional lymph nodes and Kupffer cells in the liver, and finally the macrophages in the lungs. This interaction promotes the clearance of bacteria and their toxic products, which represents the best effective response to this endogenous, infectious invasion and the stimulation and overproduction of humoral mediators, which can be deleterious for metabolism and organ function.

Once translocation occurs, the development of a septic state and possibly of MOF is a function of several factors: of these, the microbial load and virulence, BT duration and recurrence, the clearance activity of liver and pulmonary macrophages, and the magnitude of the host defense response and the amount of potentially dangerous mediators are the most important. Moreover, in critically ill patients there are many pathophysiological conditions that can contribute as predisposing factors, both enhancing BT and reducing the host defense ability. All these situations act in synergism and the BT must be considered the result of several and repeated insults, rather than the effect of a single factor.

For instance, mucosal atrophy (after feeding discontinuation and TPN) has been claimed to be the major cause of BT [1-3]. However, there are several situations of inactivity of the GIT not necessarily leading to pathological BT: for example, the ileal conduit for urinary diversion or prolonged TPN in non-critically ill patients or biliopancreatic bypass for morbid obesity.

Another highly significant condition, certainly implicated in the breakdown of the intestinal mucosal barrier, is splanchnic hypoperfusion both in terms of inadequate oxygen delivery and mismatch between oxygen delivery and oxygen requirements. There are several experimental and clinical studies which show that, in these situations, the rate of ATP hydrolysis exceeds the rate of ATP synthesis, with consequent activation of anaerobic glycolysis, mucosal acidosis, enzymatic failure, and eventually loss of cellular membrane integrity. The overall result is a breakdown of the gut barrier [3].

In critically ill patients, there are multifactorial elements which persistently and recurrently affect the gut and other organs. Some typical pathophysiological sequences in critically ill patients with poor prognosis are the cause of MOF: the clinical and biological complications, the type of injury and the good and the bad host response. All these events lead to tissue damage, organ dysfunction, and vital system impairment.

The relationships between disruption of the normal homeostatic mechanisms, intestinal dysfunction, impaired oxygen delivery, and impaired or uncontrolled host response are strictly associated, linked and mutually dependent, with a final autodestructive destination.

Clinical studies evaluating both BT and its relationship with the onset of sepsis and MOF have not provided unequivocal data and as of yet have not been able to give definitive conclusions. Baue [22] found that significant GIT problems occurred and contributed to MOF in a number of cardiothoracic patients. Moore et al. did not confirm portal or systemic bacteremia and endotoxemia within the first 5 days after injury, despite an eventual 30% incidence of MOF [23]. No differences in portal and systemic levels of cytokines were found in the patients who developed MOF. In trauma patients, infectious complications and outcome were not related to culture results of mesenteric lymph nodes, and BT to the mesenteric lymph nodes does not seem to be a common occurrence in acutely injured patients [24, 25].

Brathwaite et al. [25] showed that BT occurs in humans after traumatic injury and may be independent of hemorrhagic shock; culture techniques may not detect BT since organisms may have been phagocytized by macrophages.

Even considering the various hypotheses, there is unquestionably a relationship between translocation and MOF. In patients at risk of MOF, the GIT function is altered; gut failure and translocation are part of MOF, and many conditions can improve the bacterial and endotoxin passage through the intestinal wall. Furthermore, there are several reports confirming that GIT function is severely altered in critically ill patients [13]. In fact, during MOF, there are several anatomical and functional alterations of the GIT, such as stress ulceration, mucosal acidosis, failure of pH control in the stomach, pancreatitis, ileus and intolerance to enteral feeding, jaundice and cholestasis.

Our final remarks address the major role of the macrophage and of the whole immune system [26]. This is can be affected by several factors, including nutrition, immunologic activity, perfusion, and oxygenation, and the outcome seems to depend on the ability to show a normal response (recovery from infection), an excessive response (SIRS) or a deficient response, which leads to systemic bacteremia and MOF.

Prevention of Translocation-Prevention of MOF

Since we do not have definitive clinical data regarding BT and development of MOF, we might at least consider whether prevention of translocation can prevent systemic infection, organ dysfunction, and subsequent death. Prevention of BT can be obtained both by improving the intestinal function and the host defense mechanism [2, 3, 7].

The most reliable therapies include nutrition and early enteral feeding, selective digestive decontamination (SDD), efforts to increase oxygen delivery and to avoid tissue hypoperfusion, control of the mediator cascade and antioxidants, and improving microcirculatory blood flow. Recently, growth factors have been used to improve GIT mucosal barrier function.

The goal of nutritional support is to maintain adequate protein-caloric intake and to enable all of the critical organ functions to be carried out under circumstances of metabolic impairment. Above all, TEN is more physiological – if the gut works, use it –, although some authors consider gut dysfunction in acute stress illness to be a contraindication for TEN. Enteral feeding prevents intestinal mucosa atrophy, stimulates bile flow, promotes peristalsis and bacterial clearance, and supplies substrates not available by the parenteral route. Furthermore, in experimental studies additional glutamine in the enteral diet seems to improve nitrogen balance and intestinal mucosal cellularity [27].

The contribution of GIT infection to the high risk of septic complications in malnourished patients has not been defined. BT and death from sepsis are enhanced in malnourished animals, and bacterial adherence to mucosal epithelial cells is also increased. Patients who receive TEN following surgery or trauma have fewer septic complications than those receiving total parenteral nutrition (TPN). TEN prevents mucosal atrophy, attenuates injury stress response, maintains immunocompétence and preserves normal flora. These differences may be further magnified if the gut mucosa is malnourished from the outset. The data suggest that in malnourished patients an impairment in gut function is present and that the barrier defect becomes more generalized to a variety of antigens with progressive malnutrition. In fact, there is no specific correlation with the presence of cancer or GIT disease, suggesting that it is malnutrition per se rather than the disease which causes the alteration in barrier function. It is possible, however, that once initiated, barrier breakdown may be a factor promoting further malnutrition.

A metabolic, immunologic, and clinical improvement has been noted in patients after surgery using TEN with supplemental arginine, RNA and omega-3 fatty acids [27]. In a recent prospective study we saw an increase in hepatic protein and cholesterol synthesis in patients treated by combined enteral-parenteral nutrition versus TPN (of course, using the same calories and percentage of lipids and proteins) and a reduction in catabolic indices (urea and orotic acid excretion), with an overall lower mortality but without any statistically significant difference in the incidence of MOF.

The two most recent meta-analyses of randomized SDD-trials show significant reductions in mortality of 20% and 30%, respectively [19, 20]. Selective decontamination of the digestive tract is now an evidence-based medicine (EBM) intervention and these meta-analyses show conclusively that SDD saves lives among the critically ill [28]. The relation between infection and mortality being weak, the mechanism for benefit is high likely the significant reduction in gut endotoxin following the eradication of gut overgrowth using SDD. A reduction in gut endotoxin is associated with significantly less endotoxin absorption and is subsequently followed by recovery of systemic immunity.

A constant and adequate perfusion and oxygen delivery is essential for organ function and for preventing metabolic abnormalities. Organ dysfunction is very often related to a mismatch between oxygen demand and oxygen supply: this functional alteration becomes more evident in ischemia/reperfusion syndrome. In these circumstances there is a generation, mediated by xanthine-oxidase activity, of oxygen free radicals, followed by lipid peroxidation, Thiol and NAD depletion, and inhibition of ATP synthesis. As a consequence, new channels are formed through the membranes, which together with the dysfunction of ATP-ase, determine an increase in intracellular calcium, activation of proteases and phospholipases, and eventually cellular damage.

The use of xanthine-oxidase inhibitors and other antioxidants is consistent with these findings. Moreover, in low-flow states some authors have proposed the intraluminal administration of glucose or oxygen.

Recently, some studies claimed a beneficial effect of several growth factors on GIT barrier function. Hyuang et al [29] showed in a rat model of burn injury, that the administration of insulin-like growth factor 1 reduced gut atrophy and BT; Gianotti and co-workers [30], in a similar experimental model, demonstrated a reduction in BT using simultaneously a fibroblast growth factor and sucralfate.

The control of the mediator cascade (use of monoclonal antibodies and receptor antagonist proteins against cytokines, other mediators, and adhesion molecules) is part of the general treatment of sepsis and MOF and represents a revolution in therapeutic manipulation of the inflammatory system although it is still under investigation.

Conclusions

Considering the current state of research in this field, it is very difficult to offer definitive conclusions. BT seems to play a certain role clinically, at least in immunocompromised patients.

Most of the therapeutic strategies against translocation aim to improve the systemic nutritional and immunological status, to restore peripheral oxygen supply, to avoid hypoperfusion, to contrast anatomical intestinal mucosa defects, and prevent bacterial overgrowth. In summary, these therapeutic procedures fit with the overall clinical objectives, which are the control of tissue injury, the improvement of organ dysfunction, and eventually a positive effect on outcome.

At the present time, although the hypothesis of BT as a trigger of MOF has not been proven, we believe that the treatment of this phenomenon, if clinically relevant, has to be multifactorial with beneficial effects on the whole organism and on survival. Of course, as for several other hypotheses, more experimental and particularly clinical studies are necessary in order to make any further exhaustive conclusions on the pathophysiology of multiple organ dysfunction and to establish more effective therapies.

References

1. Gullo A, Berlot G, Silvestri L, Sganga G (1992) Sepsis and organ failure. Systems Editore, Milano
2. Sganga G, Gangeri G, Castagneto M (1998) The gut: a central organ in the development of multiple organ system failure. In: van Saene HKF, Silvestri L, de la Cal MA (eds) Infection control in the intensive care unit. Springer-Verlag, Berlin Heidelberg New York, pp 257-268
3. Sganga G, Castagneto M (1999) Bacterial translocation. In: Guarnieri G, Iscra F (eds) Metabolism and artificial nutrition in the critically ill. Springer-Verlag, Berlin Heidelberg New York, pp 203-210
4. Deich EA, Specian RD, Grisham MD (1992) Zymosan-induced bacterial translocation: a study of mechanism. Crit Care Med 20:782-786
5. Warren HS, Danner RL, Munford RS (1992) Anti-endotoxin monoclonal antibodies. N Engl J Med 326:1153-1157
6. Vincent JL, Anaissie E, Bruining H et al (1998) Epidemiology, diagnosis and treatment of systemic Candida infection in surgical patients under intensive care. Intensive Care Med 24:206-216
7. Sganga G, Gangeri G, Montemagno S, Castagneto M (1994) Prevention of translocation-prevention of multiple organ system failure. In: Mutz NJ, Koller W, Benzer H (eds) Proceedings of the 7th European Congress on Intensive Care Medicine. Monduzzi, Bologna, pp 93-101
8. Moore FA (2000) Common mucosal immunity: a novel hypothesis. Ann Surg 231:9-10
9. Moore FA (2000) The role of the gastrointestinal tract in postinjury multiple organ failure. Am J Surg (in press)
10. Moore FA, Feliciano DV, Andrassy RJ (1992) Early enteral feeding, compared with parenteral, reduces postoperative septic complications. Ann Surg 216:172-183
11. Craven DE, Kunches LM, Lichtenberg DA (1988) Nosocomial infection and fatality in medical and surgical intensive care unit patients. Arch Intern Med 148:1161-1168

12. Kanwar S, Windsor ACJW, Welsh F et al (2000) Lack of correlation between failure of gut barrier function and septic complications after major upper gastrointestinal surgery. Ann Surg 231:88-95
13. Madera JL (1990) Pathobiology of the intestinal epithelial barrier. Am J Pathol 137:1273-1279
14. Goris R (1985) MOF: generalized autodistructive inflammation. Arch Surg 120:1109-1113
15. Alexander JW, Boyce ST, Babcok GF (1990) The process of microbial translocation. Ann Surg 212:496-502
16. Deitch EA (1990) The role of intestinal barrier failure and bacterial translocation in the development of systemic and multiple organ failure. Arch Surg 125:403-406
17. Epstein MD, Banducci DR, Manders EK (1992) The role of the gastrointestinal tract in the development of burn sepsis. Plast Reconstr Surg 90:524-529
18. Deitch EA (1992) Multiple organ failure. Pathophysiology and potential future therapy. Ann Surg 216:117-134
19. D'amico R, Pifferi S, Leonetti V et al (1988) Effectiveness of antibiotic prophylaxis in critically ill adult patients: systematic review of randomized controlled trials. BMJ 316:1275-1285
20. Nathens AB, Marshall JC (1999) Selective decontamination of the digestive tract in surgical patients. A systematic review of the evidence. Arch Surg 134:170-176
21. van Saene HKF, Silvestri L, de la Cal M (2000) Prevention of nosocomial infections in the intensive care unit. Curr Opin Crit Care 6:323-329
22. Baue AE (1993) The role of the gut in the development of multiple organ dysfunction. Ann Thorac Surg 55:822-828
23. Moore FA, Moore EE, Poggetti R et al (1991) Gut bacterial translocation via the portal vein: a clinical perspective with major torso trauma. J Trauma 31:629-636
24. Peitzman AB, Udekwu AO, Ochoa J, Smith S (1991) Bacterial translocation in trauma patients. J Trauma 31:1083-1086
25. Brathwaite CEM, Ross SE, Nagele R (1993) Translocation occurs in humans after traumatic injury: evidence using immunofluorescence. J Trauma 34:586-590
26. Wells CL, Maddaus MA, Simmons RL (1987) Role of the macrophage in the translocation of intestinal bacteria. Arch Surg 122:48-54
27. Daly JM, Lieberman MD (1992) Enteral nutrition with supplemental arginine, RNA and omega-3 fatty acids in patients after operation: immunologic, metabolic, and clinical outcome. Surgery 112:56-61
28. Silvestri L, Mannucci F, van Saene HKF (2000) Selective decontamination of the digestive tract: a life-saver. J Hosp Infect 45:185-190
29. Hyuang KF, Chung DH, Herndon DN (1993) Insulinlike growth factor reduces gut atrophy and bacterial translocation after severe burn injury. Arch Surg 128:47-53
30. Gianotti L, Alexander W, Jukushima R, Pyles T (1993) Reduction of bacterial translocation with oral fibroblast growth factor and sucralfate. Am J Surg 165:195-201

Chapter 6

Practical Aspects of Antibiotic Prophylaxis in High-Risk Surgical Patients

G. Sganga, G. Brisinda, M. Castagneto

Introduction

Infection is the most important complication of surgical procedures, and it continues to be a disconcerting cause of death in surgical patients. Postoperative infections, too, increase morbidity and prolong hospitalization [1]. Surgical patients can develop several postoperative infections; wound infection – representing more than 19% of all postoperative infections – is the most common, but also respiratory tract infections (14%), urinary tract infections (13%), fever of unknown etiology (7%), and thrombophlebitis (2.5%) are important causes of postoperative morbidity. These complications add 10%-20% additional costs to the total hospital bill [1]. In the United States, for any given type of operation, the development of a wound infection will approximately double the cost of hospitalization. Proper antibiotic prophylaxis reduces these costs.

On the other hand, inappropriate and indiscriminate use of antibiotics in the perioperative period can increase costs and select resistant organisms [2-4].

As with other adjunctive measure in surgery, proper antibiotic prophylaxis is not a substitute for excellent patient care, such as good operative technique, appropriate infection control practice, patient preparation, and operating environment. Furthermore, antibiotic prophylaxis is a primary factor that should be considered in preparing the patient for surgery.

The goals of proper antibiotic prophylaxis in surgery are to prevent wound infection and deep abscess, mainly intra-abdominal abscess, caused by intraoperative bacterial contamination [5]. On the other hand, treatment of an already existing infection is a matter of therapy, not of prophylaxis.

To date, most studies showing a clear-cut benefit from such antibiotics have involved surgical procedures that bore an appreciable risk of infection (Tab. 1). Furthermore, multiple clinical trials showed that systemic antibiotics are highly effective when used just before, during, and immediately after an operation.

In this review, we summarize the recent knowledge on surgical infections and practical aspects of antibiotic prophylaxis in high-risk surgical patients.

Wound Infections

Infection of the wound is a very frequent event after a surgical procedure. A simple method for evaluating the probability that a wound infection will develop consists in classifying the wound according to the scheme illustrated in Tab. 2.

Table 1. Surgical procedures in which systemic antibiotic prophylaxis is of benefit

- Head and neck surgery, which require opening the upper aerodigestive tract
- Esophageal, excluding hiatal hernia repair
- Gastroduodenal, except for complications of uncorrected hyperacidity
- Biliary tract for patients aged more 70 years, with acute cholecystitis, and/or requiring choledochostomy
- Small and large bowel resections
- Anorectal procedures
- Appendecectomy for gangrenous or perforated appendix
- Hysterectomy
- Abdominal and lower extremity revascularizations, including prostethic grafts
- Other clean surgical procedures implanting high-risk prostheses, e.g. hip, knee, aortic valve

Risk Factors for Wound Infections

Surgical wound infections occur whenever the combination of microbial numbers and the virulence in the wound is sufficiently large to overcome the local host defense mechanisms and progressive growth is established. It is immediately evident that different types of surgical procedures, involving a greater or lesser degree of contamination and dissection, are then associated with different probabilities of developing wound infections. For hernia repair [6] or thyroidectomy, the probabil-

Table 2. Classification of surgical wounds according to risk of infection

Type	Definition
Clean	When no contamination is present • Nontraumatic • No break in technique • Respiratory, digestive or genitourinary tracts not entered
Clean-contaminated	When no significant contamination is present • Gastrointestinal or respiratory tract entered without significant spillage • Oropharynx, vagina or noninfected genitourinary or biliary tract entered • Minor break in technique
Contaminated	When there is inflammation and/or gross contamination • Major break in technique • Traumatic wound • Gross spillage from the gastrointestinal tract • Entrance into infected genitourinary or biliary tracts
Dirty or infected	When pus is present or in presence of a perforated viscus

ity of wound infection is very low, about 2% or even less. For cholecystectomy or hysterectomy about 6% and for gastrointestinal procedures such as partial colectomy, subtotal gastric resection, or appendectomy it is about 11%. Nephrectomies and radical mastectomies carry a high probability of wound infection, in the neighborhood of 15%, because of the large dissection in often elderly suffering from neoplastic primary diseases [7, 8].

The dependency of the infection rate on the type of surgery is reflected in the overall differences in infection rates to be expected in the different departments of surgery, from a low of 2% in plastic surgery, to 3-5% in orthopaedics, gynaecology and vascular surgery, to a high of 8 to 10% in general surgery and urology [1]. Moreover, the fact that different surgeons in the same department often have widely different infection rates underscores the importance of surgical technique in the prevention of infection.

Several patient factors, besides the type of procedure and the skill of the operator, are important in affecting the probability of incurring a postoperative wound infection. One important factor is the age of the patient: the higher the age, the higher the incidence, from less than 1% in teens to more than 3% in seniors, overall. Another factor is the period of hospital stay before surgery: patients hospitalized for more than 12 days are more liable to develop an infected wound, showing that a relationship is likely to exist between the incidence of infection and the hospital environment and bacterial flora.

Factors Involved in Development of Wound Infections

It is clear that the mechanism whereby a patient develops a wound infection is linked to three critical elements. These are represented by the closed space, the infectious agent, which must be present in sufficient numbers and with sufficient virulence, and the susceptible host.

Injury produces enclosed environments without ready access to oxygen and immune cells and molecules via a number of mechanisms: pockets of extravasated blood, dead tissue, infarcted areas, natural spaces, foreign bodies, and prostheses. The environment in these enclosed spaces becomes soon hypoxic, hypercarbic, and acidic, favoring bacterial growth. In abdominal surgery, the gastrointestinal tract represents a huge reservoir of pathogenic bacteria. Recently it has been hypothesized that the gastrointestinal tract could act as an undrained abscess, causing infection and multiple organ dysfunction.

Any infectious agent can contaminate a closed space, but relatively few cause infection. Streptococci invade even minor breaks in the skin and spread through connective tissue planes and lymphatics. Staphylococci are less invasive but more pathogenic. *Pseudomonas* and *Serratia* are seen most frequently as opportunistic invaders. Many fungi and parasites may cause abscesses or sinus and are typical of the immunocompromised patient. Anaerobes (Bacteroides) and peptostreptococci are more frequently isolated because of improvements in culture techniques. Post-surgical infection is a multimicrobial disease and, unfortunately, many bacteria act in synergism.

Finally, there are host-dependent, predisposing factors to the development of post-surgical infection. Among these are diabetes, severe trauma, burns, malnutrition, cancer, hematologic disorders, transplantation, and immunosuppressive drugs. In many patients, these factors are believed to be primarily responsible for a decreased reactivity to delayed hypersensitivity antigens, creating an anergic state associated with an increased incidence of infectious complications [9]. However, more patients with a high susceptibility to infection are now subjected to surgery than was the case even a few years ago.

Considering these three elements, it is easier to understand the vicious cycle that many times we have to confront: in a surgical patient, it is very common to find a certain degree of immunosuppression and anergy; anergy leads to infection, but more importantly the infection itself can deteriorate the immune system. Our role is to oppose the development of this vicious cycle by physiologic support: nutritional support, antibiotics, and surgical drainage.

The importance of the nutritional status is emphasized by the higher incidence of infections and other surgical complications in malnourished patients. Among several nutritional status indices, the prognostic nutritional index (PNI), which explicitly includes the serum albumin value, has been shown to be correlated with the probability of infection after surgery. A high risk of postoperative complications has been found to correspond to values of PNI above 50%; an intermediate risk to values between 40 and 49%; and a low risk to values below 40%.

The overall result of the altered host factors is a decreased efficiency of the mechanisms and systems essential for host defense. The components of the host defense system are the skin and mucous membranes, the phagocytes, the reticuloendothelial system, humoral and cellular immunity, complement, and acute phase proteins. Alterations in these components, once induced, may persist for up to 1 month. The cellular, vascular and humoral components of the inflammatory response depend on these elements, with the goal of achieving a reduction in cellular damage and the resolution of infection.

Antibiotic Prophylaxis

Since infectious complications in surgical patients are responsible for prolonged wound healing, disability, deformity, and even death, and since the patient's quality of life can be affected or even permanently altered by them, including very high human and economic costs, it is important to prevent them as far as possible.

We can do this by improving the patient's ability to oppose the microorganism invasion, by good surgical procedure, and by using antibiotic prophylaxis.

The first important point about antibiotic prophylaxis is administration timing [1, 5, 10]. It has been shown that administration of antibiotics just before, during, and up to 3 h after surgery effectively prevents wound infections. Many experimental and clinical studies demonstrated that prophylactic antibiotics are most useful if given to patients before contamination has occurred [10]. Typical pioneer studies investigated the diameter of lesions induced by staphylococcal inoculation and the effect of timed penicillin administration: the most relevant protective effect was observed when antibiotic was given 1 h before staphylococcal inoculation and the protection decreased rapidly if the penicillin was administered later.

Antibiotic must be given so that good tissue levels are present at the time of the procedure and for the first 3-4 h after the surgical incision. There is little evidence supporting the prophylactic action of antibiotics past the period of operation and recovery of normal physiology following anesthesia. A practical approach would then contemplate administering a single preoperative dose, followed by an intra-operative dose in case of prolonged procedures.

Principles of proper prophylaxis of wound infections include the selection of bactericidal antibiotics effective against likely pathogens. Studies have shown that single agent prophylaxis is almost always effective in the majority of clinical situations, provided that the half-life of antibiotic is long enough to maintain adequate tissue levels throughout the operation and that the dose is equal to a full therapeutic intravenous dose [11].

From the practical point of view, the antibiotic should be administered immediately before skin incision. A second dose should be given only if the procedure lasts longer than 3 h (or twice the half-life of the antibiotic) or massive hemorrhage has occurred during surgery. Postoperative doses are generally unnecessary and are not warranted beyond 24 h.

Recommended antibiotics for prophylaxis of wound infections caused by gram-positive and gram-negative aerobic bacteria are cefazolin 1 i.v./i.m. or vancomycin 1 i.v. in patients allergic to cephalosporins. First-generation cephalosporins (such as cefazolin) are a good choice because they are not expensive, have not shown a low rate of allergic responses, and have a broad spectrum of activity against likely aerobic pathogens.

Prophylaxis against both gram-negative aerobes and anaerobes includes clindamycin (or metronidazole) plus tobramycin, or a single broad-spectrum agent such as cefoxitin or cefotetan or sulbactam/amipicillin. Gram-negative anaerobes (Bacteroides species) originate in the intestine and are synergistic with gram-negative aerobes in causing infections after abdominal/intestinal surgical procedures. Even though the problem is still a matter of debate, there is evidence that the antibiotic treatment in these infections should be directed against both aerobic and anaerobic agents. The combination of two antibiotics (clindamycin, metronidazole are specific against gram-negative anaerobes; the amynoglicoside against gram-negative aerobes) is in general more powerful than a single broad-spectrum agent active against both bacterial components (i.e., cefoxitin, cefotetan, imipenem, sulbactam/ampicillin). Clinical studies have shown that, in cases of colorectal surgery with anastomotic leakage, the overall infection rates without therapy are of the order of 10%, those with therapy of only 4%. These data very clearly demonstrate that the infection rate after colorectal surgery is much lower by using an antibiotic regimen against aerobes and anaerobes in comparison to no treatment.

A second point concerns the cases for which antibiotic prophylaxis as described is indicated. In general, an approach such as that outlined above is indicated for gastrointestinal and anorectal surgery, biliary tract surgery, vaginal hysterectomy, insertion of artificial devices such as cardiovascular or hip-joint prostheses, or for prolonged clean surgery (more than 3 h in duration). This indication is then valid in general for clean-contaminated surgery or for surgery contemplating the use of prostheses. In contaminated or dirty surgery the case is different, and we have to consider appropriate therapy, which should be started as soon as possible and continued for 2-3 days.

The overall criteria for any antibiotic therapy are that it must be safe with low toxicity; it must be active against the suspected pathogens; it should contemplate a short course of therapy; and it should be used as perioperative treatment only in immunocompromised patients or patients with severe infections.

In relation to operative contamination and increasing risk of infection, the classification of operative wounds includes four categories, mentioned above in Table 2. This is the most widely applied classification of surgical procedures in terms of contamination and probability that a wound infection will develop; this risk is about 5%, 10%, 15% and 30% for the four reported classes, respectively.

Clean Wounds

Clean wounds have an infection risk of about 1.5%-4.2%. Prophylactic antibiotics are not indicated in clean operation if the patient does not have host-risk factors.

Factors suggesting the need for prophylaxis are remote infection, diabetes, and at least three concomitant medically diagnosed conditions. Additive risk factors are, also, abdominal operations and operations expected to last longer than 2 h.

Prostheses implants are clean procedures, some of which require antibiotic prophylaxis. Heart valves, vascular grafts, orthopaedic implants necessitate prophylaxis with either cefazolin or vancomycin. In contrast, catheters (vascular, peritoneal), pacemakers and shunts are at very low risk of infection so that prophylaxis is usually not necessary, according to our experience. Inguinal hernia repair with biomaterials does not benefit from antibiotic prophylaxis [12, 13].

Clean-Contaminated Wounds

Clean-contaminated wounds are at 10% risk of infection or lower. Clean-contaminated surgery usually requires prophylaxis [1, 5, 13].

Contaminated Wounds

Contaminated wounds are at 10%-20% risk of infection. This type of surgery requires prophylaxis [1,5].

Head and neck, gynaecological, and urologic procedures are usually clean-contaminated cases. If the operation involves entry in the oral/digestive cavity, cefazolin (or clindamycin) is recommended [14]. High-risk caesarean section, abortion, and vaginal or abdominal hysterectomy require cefazolin (or doxycycline, or cefoxitin). In urologic procedures in patients with positive urine cultures, the right choice is a single dose of sensitive antibiotic for prophylaxis.

Biliary, hepatobiliary, and pancreatic operations usually meet criteria of the definition of clean-contaminated wounds. In biliary tract procedures prophylaxis is required only for cases at high risk of contamination: bile obstruction, jaundice, stones in common duct, reoperation, and cholecystitis. A single dose of cefazolin is recommended. Prophylaxis (with cefazolin) is always required in hepatobiliary and pancreatic surgery because these intra-abdominal operations are long.

In gastroduodenal operations the risk is low if gastric acidity is normal and bleeding, cancer, gastric ulcer and obstruction are absent. No prophylaxis is warranted. All other patients are at high risk of infections and a single dose of cefazolin is appropriate. In surgery for morbid obesity the dose of cefazolin should be doubled.

Colorectal procedures usually represent contaminated cases. The unique goals of prophylaxis include the preoperative reduction of fecal mass and of bacteria concentration in feces. Mechanical bowel preparation is successfully obtained with the technique of whole gut lavage (PEG - polyethylene glycole solutions) the day before surgery. On the same day, oral antibiotics active against both aerobes and anaerobes are given in order to reduce bacterial concentration in feces [15]. Typically, they are rapidly bactericidal, poorly absorbed, and non toxic: neomycin or kanamycin, plus erythromycin or metronidazole 1 g each is the usual choice.

The timing of antibiotic administration is critical. If given earlier, they may not be useful or can produce resistance. Parenteral broad-spectrum antibiotics are considered optional because the orally given agents reach usually therapeutic levels in tissues. However, parenteral antibiotics are reported to further reduce the postoperative infection rate [16]. Cefoxitin, or cefotetan, or clindamycin (or metronidazole) plus gentamicin are used in a single dose just before surgery.

Appendectomy only requires parenteral single-agent (or combination) administration, active against both aerobes and anaerobes. If the infection is surgically removed, prophylaxis is adequate; othewise antibiotic administration is repeated as therapy.

Bowel preparation (mechanical plus oral antibiotics) is used in major elective abdominal procedures (i.e., vascular graft) to prevent bacterial translocation from the gut possibly related to low-state flow in intestinal perfusion during surgical procedure.

Infected Wounds

Dirty and infected wounds (risk of infection 20%-40%) meet the following criteria: acute bacterial inflammation, without pus; transection of clean tissue for the purpose of surgical access to a collection of pus; traumatic wound with retained ischemic tissues; foreign bodies; fecal contamination; or delayed treatment. The right treatment is to administer antibiotic therapy, not as prophylaxis, because infection is already present.

However, there are several particular clinical situations that may belong to the category of dirty cases.

For instance, a laparotomy can be performed without precise preoperative diagnosis. It is usually an emergency procedure and demands prophylaxis with cefazolin. Suspected ruptured viscus requires an agent (or combination) active against both aerobes and anaerobes. If rupture is found, antibiotics are administered as therapy.

Trauma can be a clean or clean-contaminated or contaminated or dirty case, but at the moment of first aid the categorization could be unclear. The sequela of an infection can be severe in trauma patients; then antibiotic prophylaxis is adequate. The administration should be given early and then considered an integral part of resuscitation of the patient [17]. The proper duration of prophylaxis remains unclear (24-48 h or less, according to different studies).

Recommended antibiotics are cefoxitin or a combination of agents active against both aerobes and anaerobes in abdominal injury, cefazolin in open fractures (usually as a therapeutic course), and in major soft tissue injury.

Prophylaxis of endocarditis is frequently required in the critically ill patient. The rationale is to treat transient bacteremia during endoscopic or minor surgical procedures: dental or oropharyngeal, respiratory (bronchoscopy), urologic, and gastrointestinal (endoscopy, biopsies, sclerotherapy). The most common bacteria involved are *Streptococcus viridans* and *Enterococcus*, the former in dental/respiratory procedures, the latter in the gastrointestinal or genitourinary tract.

Oral amoxicillin (3 g before the procedure, then 1.5 g 6 h later) is a proper prophylaxis against *Streptococcus viridans*. Erythromycin or clindamycin are good substitutes. *Enterococcus* can be treated with ampicillin (2 g i.v. before the procedure, then 1.5 g 6 h later) plus gentamicin, or with vancomycin plus gentamicin.

Selective Decontamination of the Digestive Tract

Antibiotic prophylaxis includes the selective decontamination of the digestive tract (SDD) in critically ill patients admitted to ICU. Previous studies demonstrated that bacterial colonization of the oropharynx and gastrointestinal tract by hospital-acquired pathogens is the major source of endogenous infection (mainly respiratory) in patients undergoing mechanical ventilation. Nonabsorbable topical antibiotics applied to the oropharynx and instilled in the stomach have been shown to reduce both morbidity and mortality by 65% an 20%, respectively [18-21]. The benefits were even greater in a meta-analysis of randomized SDD trials in which more than 70% of the enrolled patients were surgical. Pneumonia and mortality were reduced by 80% and 30%, respectively [19].

Debated indications of SDD are related to its action in preventing endotoxin translocation during intestinal ischemia or in liver insufficiency. Experiments in rats with sterile peritonitis showed that SDD prevents translocation of gram-negative bacilli to the abdominal cavity, endotoxemia, and mortality [22].

In liver transplant patients SDD proved able to reduce gram-negative pulmonary colonization and respiratory infections but not systemic endotoxemia and organ system failure [23].

During cardiopulmonary bypass, previously administered SDD eliminated enterobacteria from the gut and prevented peroperative increases in serum endo-toxin and activation of cytokines [24, 25].

Nonsurgical Infections in Surgical Patients

Rates of nosocomial pneumonia seem to be higher in critically ill surgical patients than in patients admitted to a medical ICU, and the mortality attributable to noso-comial pneumonia is notably greater in the surgical sub-population [26]. Pulmonary infection has been shown to be independent risk factor for mortality in patients with abdominal sepsis [27]. These data are in line with the Canadian meta-analysis of surgical SDD-trials, showing that surgical patients may benefit more from SDD compared with medical patients [19].

Superinfection

A superinfection is an infection that develops during antibiotic treatment for a previous infection. The superinfection rate varies between 2%-10% of antibiotic-treated patients.

Antibiotics exert a selective pressure on the patient's flora [28] and may subsequently lead to the emergence of micro-organisms resistant to the antibiotic. Practically all superinfections are due to multi-resistant micro-organisms. Respiratory tract infections are common superinfections occurring during the treatment of intra-abdominal infection [27].

Antibiotic-associated colitis is another significant superinfection that can occur in hospitalized patients with mild to severe illness. This entity is caused by *Clostridium difficile*, an enteric pathogen, and can vary from a self-limited, mild disease to a rapidly progressive septic process, often culminating in death.

Fungal infections are most common in patients with neutropenia and cancer; however, it has been recognized that the incidence of *Candida* infections is increasing in critically ill patients without the latter conditions. Furthermore, the rates of *Candida* spp bloodstream infections have increased markedly during the past decade: a fivefold increase in nosocomial bloodstream infection rates has been observed between 1980 and 1989 [29], the greatest increase occurring in surgical patients; in recent years the patient population admitted to the ICU has changed, the number of patients receiving immunosoppressive antineoplastic or antirejection therapies has grown, and the improvements in supportive care have created a group of long-term ICU residents at risk of fungal infection.

Furthermore, the use of broad-spectrum antibacterial agents seems to be particularly important: their suppression of gastrointestinal flora allows the proliferation of *Candida* within the gut, which predisposes to systemic infection. Although the pathogenesis of systemic candidiasis is not completely understood, the likely initial step is patient colonization. This is an independent risk factor for candidemia [30] and predisposes to the development of subsequent severe infections in patients recovering from abdominal surgery. A role for colonization was suggested earlier, in 1972 [31]. Solomkin et al. highlighted the role of the intensity of the colonization process in the development of candidemia in surgical patients [32]. The authors also suggested that early antifungal therapy may be beneficial in patients colonized at more than two sites, but without candidemia. Other studies on patients recovering from abdominal surgery have indicated that *Candida* spp isolation in pure culture might constitute an indication for antifungal therapy [33]. Moreover, the use of broad-spectrum antibiotics promoting *Candida* spp proliferation in the gastrointestinal tract was identified as an independent risk factor for infection. This use increases the risk for acquiring fungal infections, and fungal overgrowth typically complicates antimicrobial treatments, but opinions differ about its clinical significance. Previously, it was shown that the type and number of antibiotics predicted infections; recent findings add to these observations because both the length of antimicrobial therapy before the beginning of fungal colonization ($p = 0.03$) and before infection ($p < 0.02$) were shown to be associated significantly with subsequent *Candida* infection. These results reinforce the conviction that an effective restrictive antibiotic policy may be one of the most important care standards for preventing life-threatening infections [34, 35] and also strongly re-emphazises the importance of discontinuing antibiotic treatment as early as possible in critically ill patients.

The difficulty in treating these patients is distinguishing colonization with *Candida* from invasive infection. Multiple surveillance cultures are performed daily in critically ill patients, but the clinical importance of positive *Candida* spp cultures has not been defined; no current recommendation exists for initiating therapy based on the degree of colonization. The diagnosis of severe fungal infection may be difficult, although the clinical conditions which predispose patients to these infections are becoming better known and more effective therapies are increasingly available.

Deciding when to initiate antifungal therapy is often troublesome, due to the difficulty to detect disseminated infection. Those patients who are candidemic require therapy, but some patients with systemic infection may have negative blood cultures. Given the high mortality associated with candidemia, early presumptive antifungal therapy should be considered in patients who are at high risk of *Candida* infection. The use of fluconazole as early presumptive therapy in ICU patients is an area in which well-designed clinical studies are urgently required. Furthermore, systemic antifungal prophylaxis is not recommended in the surgical ICU population. Some centers use prophylaxis in liver transplant recipients, and fluconazole or amphotericin B is added to the regimens used prior to surgery.

References

1. Howard RJ, Simmons RL (1988) Surgical infectious diseases. Appleton and Lange, Norwalk
2. Page CP, Bohnen J, Fletcher R et al (1993) Antimicrobial prophylaxis for surgical wounds. Arch Surg 128:79-88
3. Leaper DJ (1994) Prophylactic and therapeutic role of the antibiotics in wound care. Am J Surg 167:15-20

4. Scher KS, Bernstein JM, Arenstein GL, Sorensen C (1990) Reducing the cost of surgical prophylaxis. Am Surg 56:32-35
5. Sganga G, De Gaetano A, Gangeri G, Castagneto M (1991) Antibiotic strategies in intra-abdominal sepsis. In Gullo A (Ed) Recent advances in anaesthesia pain intensive care and emergency. APICE, Trieste, pp 575-580
6. Gilbert AI, Felton LL (1993) Infection in inguinal hernia repair considering biomaterials and antibiotics. Surg Gynecol Obst 177:126-30
7. Dunn DL (2000) Diagnosis and treatment of infection. In: Norton JA, Bollinger RR, Chang AE, Lowry SF, Mulvihill SJ, Pass HI Thompson RW (eds) Surgery. Basic science and clinical evidence. Springer-Verlag New York, 193-220
8. Pollock AV (1990) The treatment of infected wounds. Acta Chir Scand 156:505-513
9. Delves PJ, Roitt IM (2000) Advances in immunology: the immune system. N Engl J Med 343:37-49
10. Classen DC, Evans RS, Pestotnik A (1992) The timing of prophylactic administration of antibiotics and the risk of surgical-wound infection. N Engl J Med 326:281-287
11. Citak MS, Cue JL, Peyton JC, Malangoni MA (1992) The critical relationship of antibiotic dose and bacterial contamination in experimental infection. J Surg Res 52:127-130
12. Gilbert Al, Felton LL (1993) Infection in inguinal hernia repair considering biomaterials and antibiotics. Surg Gynecol Obstet 177:126-131
13. Hulten L (1994) Dressings for surgical wounds. Am J Surg 67:428-458
14. Velanovich V (1991) A meta-analysis of prophylactic antibiotics in head and neck surgery. Plast Reconstr Surg 87:429-434
15. Nichols RL (1984) Update on preparation of the colon for resection. Current Surg 41:75-82
16. Coppa GF, Eng K, Gouge TH (1983) Parenteral and oral antibiotics in elective colon and rectal surgery: a prospective and randomized trial. Am J Surg 145:62-67
17. Reed RL, Ericsson CD, Wu A et al (1992) The pharmacokinetics of prophylactic antibiotics in trauma. J Trauma 32:21-27
18. D'Amico R, Pifferi S, Leonetti V et al (1998) Effectiveness of antibiotic prophylaxis in critically ill adult patients: systematic review of randomised controlled trials. BMJ 316:1275-1285
19. Nathens AB, Marshall JC (1999) Selective decontamination of the digestive tract in surgical patients. A systematic review of the evidence. Arch Surg 134:170-176
20. Silvestri L, Mannucci F, van Saene HKF (2000) Selective decontamination of the digestive tract: a life-saver. J Hosp Infect 45:185-190
21. Van Saene HKF, Silvestri L, de la Cal M (2000) Prevention of nosocomial infections in the intensive care unit. Curr Opin Crit Care 6:323-329
22. Rosman C, Wubbels GH, Manson WL, Bleichrodt RP (1992) Selective decontamination of the digestive tract prevents secondary infection of the abdominal cavity and endotoxemia and mortality in sterile peritonitis in laboratory rats. Crit Care Med 20:1699-1704
23. Bion JF, Badger I, Crosby HA et al(1994) Selective decontamination of the digestive tract reduces gram-negative pulmonary colonization but not systemic edotoxemia in patients undergoing elective liver trasplantation. Crit Care Med 22:40-49
24. Martinez-Pellus AE, Merino P, Bru M et al (1993) Can selective digestive decontamination avoid the endotoxemia and cytokine activation promoted by cardiopulmonary bypass? Crit Care Med 21:1684-91
25. Martinez-Pellus AE, Merino P, Bru M et al (1997) Endogenous endotoxemia of intestinal origin during cardiopulmonary bypass. Intensive Care Med 23:1251-1257

26. Cunnion KM, Weber DJ, Broadhead WE et al (1996) Risk factors of nosocomial pneumonia: comparing adult critical-care populations. Am J Respir Crit Care Med 153:158-162

27. Mustard RA, Bohnen JMA, Rosati C et al (1991) Pneumonia complicating abdominal sepsis. Arch Surg 126:170-175

28. Sganga G, Castagneto M (1999) Bacterial translocation. In: Guarnieri G, Iscra F (eds) Metabolism and artificial nutrition in the critically ill. Springer-Verlag, Berlin Heidelberg New York, pp 203-210

29. Sganga G, Gangeri G, Montemagno S, Castagneto M (1994) Prevention of translocation – prevention of multiple organ system failure. In: Mutz NJ, Koller W, Benzer H (eds.) Proceedings of the 7th European Congress on Intensive Care Medicine. Monduzzi, Bologna, pp 93-101

30. Vincent JL, Anaissie E, Bruining H et al (1998) Epidemiology, diagnosis and treatment of systemic Candida infection in surgical patients under intensive care. Intensive Care Med 24:206-216

31. Moore FA (2000) Common mucosal immunity: a novel hypothesis. Ann Surg 231: 9-10

32. Solomkin JS, Flohr AB, Quie PG, Simmons RL (1980) The role of Candida in intraperitoneal infections. Surgery 88:524-530

33. Solomkin JS, Flohr AB, Simmons RL (1982) Indications for therapy for fungemia in postoperative patients. Arch Surg 117:1272-1275

34. Emmerson AM (1990) The epidemiology of infections in intensive care units. Intensive Care Med 16 (S3):197-200

35. Pittet D, Suter PM (1989) Judicious use of antibiotics in critically ill patients. In: Vincent JL (ed) Update in intensive care and emergency medicine, vol 8. Springer, Berlin Heidelberg New York, pp 154-163

Capitolo 7

The Usefulness of Surveillance Cultures: a Prospective Cohort Study on the ICU

H.K.F. van Saene, N. Taylor, N. Reilly, J. Hughes, K.R. Shankar, P. Baines, R. Sarginson

Surveillance Samples

Definition

Surveillance samples are defined as samples obtained from body sites where potentially pathogenic micro-organisms (PPM) are carried, i.e., the digestive tract comprising the oropharyngeal cavity and rectum [1]. Surveillance swabs are to be distinguished from surface and diagnostic samples. Surface samples are swabs from the skin such as axilla, groin and umbilicus, and from the nose, eye and ear. They do not belong to a surveillance sampling protocol, because positive surface swabs merely reflect oropharyngeal and rectal carrier state. Diagnostic samples are samples from internal organs that are normally sterile, such as lower airways, blood, bladder, and skin lesions. They are only taken on clinical indication. The endpoint of diagnostic samples is clinical, as they aim to microbiologically prove a clinical diagnosis of inflammation, both generalized and/or local.

Aim

The aim of obtaining surveillance cultures is the determination of the microbiological endpoint of the carrier state of potentially pathogenic micro-organisms [2]. Carriage or carrier state exists when the same bacterial strain is isolated from at least two consecutive surveillance samples of the ICU patient in any concentration over a period of at least 1 week. Carriage implies persistent presence of a micro-organism and is distinguished from acquisition or transient presence. Surveillance samples are not useful for diagnosing infection of lungs, blood, bladder or wounds as diagnostic samples are required for this purpose. To adhere to the definition of infection, a substantial number of leukocytes ($\geq$ ++ on a scale of; +, few; ++, moderate; +++many, or $\geq 100 \times 10^6/l$) and micro-organisms ($\geq 3+$ or $10^5/ml$) must be present in the diagnostic sample (see below).

Sampling for Surveillance Purposes

What Sites?

A throat and rectal swab are taken to detect oropharyngeal and gut carriage of aerobic Gram-negative bacilli (AGNB). For monitoring the carrier state of methicillin-resistant *Staphylococcus aureus* (MRSA), a nasal swab must be added. As MRSA has an affinity for the skin, skin is sampled only if lesions are present.

When?

Surveillance sets are obtained on admission and twice weekly thereafter (Monday, Thursday) throughout the ICU stay, in order to distinguish carriage due to potentially pathogenic micro-organisms imported in the admission flora ("import") from ICU-associated PPM acquired in nasopharynx and gut during the ICU stay ("nosocomial" or "super" carriage).

Microbiological Procedures

The target micro-organisms of surveillance samples are AGNB, methicillin-sensitive and -resistant *S. aureus* and yeasts. These potentially pathogenic micro-organisms are selected for microbiological screening, as systemic antimicrobials, in general, fail to clear carriage of these micro-organisms. The purpose of selective decontamination of the digestive tract (SDD) is to prevent or eradicate, if initially present, carriage of AGNB, *S. aureus*, and yeasts using polymyxin E, tobramycin, and amphotericin B (PTA) [3]. Oral vancomycin is only added in case of MRSA.

Throat and rectal swabs are processed qualitatively and semi-quantitatively, including an enrichment broth, to detect the level of carriage [4].

Three solid media, MacConkey (AGNB), staphylococcal, and yeast agar, are inoculated using the four quadrant method, and a brain-heart infusion broth culture is included. Each swab is streaked onto the three solid media, then the tip is broken off into 5 ml of enrichment broth. All cultures are incubated aerobically at 37°C. The MacConkey plate is examined after one night, the plates for staphylococci and yeasts after two nights. In addition, if the enrichment broth is turbid after one night's incubation, it is then inoculated onto the three media. A semi-quantitative estimation is made by grading growth density on a scale of 1+ to 5+, as follows: growth in broth only = 1+ (c. 10 microorganisms/ml), growth in the first quadrant of the solid plate = 2+ ($\geq$10^3/ml), in the second quadrant = 3+ ($\geq$10^5/ml), in the third quadrant = 4+ ($\geq$10^7/ml), and on the whole plate = 5+ ($\geq$10^9/ml). Macroscopically distinct colonies are isolated in pure culture. Standard methods for identification, typing, and sensitivity patterns are used for all microorganisms. All data are entered into the computer. A simple program enables the intensive care specialist to view the microbiological overview chart of each long-stay patient at the bedside [4] (Tabs. 1, 2).

Table. 1. Oropharyngeal and gastrointestinal carriage detected by surveillance samples is shown in combination with the colonization/infection data obtained from the diagnostic samples of lower airways, bladder, and blood. The overview chart shows that both primary and secondary endogenous infections occur after 48 h in a patient who is traditionally managed

ICU, days	1	2	3	4	5	6	7	8	9	10	11	12	13	14	15	16	17	18	19	20	21	22	23	24	25	26
Antibiotics						penicillin G									ceftazidime/amikacin											
Oropharynx																										
S. aureus	1+		2+							—			—				—			—				—		
Candida	1+		3+			4+				1+			2+				2+			1+				2+		
P. aerug										1+			3+				3+			2+				2+		
E. cloac			1+			2+																				
E. coli	1+																									
Lower airways																										
P. aerug													1+		2+	3+			1+			1+		2+		
S. pneu	1+		3+			—																				
Gut																										
S. aureus	3+		2+			2+				—			—				—			—				—		
Candida	2+		2+			3+				2+			3+				2+			1+				2+		
E. coli	4+		3+			4+				4+			2+				3+			2+				4+		
P. aerug													3+				3+			4+				3+		
Klebsiella													1+				1+			2+				3+		
E. cloac										1+			3+				3+			2+				3+		
Bladder																										
Candida	—												1+							—						
Blood																										
P. aerug																	+									
S. pneu			+																						+	

Table. 2. The microbiological chart shows the pattern of a trauma patient who received the full protocol of selective decontamination of the digestive tract, immediately on admission. Cefotaxime controlled primary endogenous infection developing within the first week, and the topical polymyxin E/tobramycin/amphotericin B (PTA) prevented the development of supercarriage and subsequent supercolonization and infection

ICU, days	1	2	3	4	5	6	7	8	9	10	11	12	13	14	15	16	17	18	19	20	21	22	23	24	25	26
Antibiotics	Cefotaxime (1–4)				Polymyxin E/tobramycin B (PTA)																					
Oropharynx																										
S. aureus	1+	2+	2+		—			—				—			—		—		—							
Candida	2+	1+	—		—			—				1+			—		—		1+							
Lower airways																										
S. aureus	1+	1+	1+	—	—			—				—			—		—		—							
Gut																										
S. aureus	3+	3+	3+		2+			2+	1+			—			1+		—		1+							
Candida	1+	—			2+			2+	3+			2+			1+		—		—							
E.coli	2+	3+	3+		2+			2+	3+			2+			—		—		—							
	—			—	—										—		—		—							
Bladder		—			—										—		—		—							
Blood		—		—	—				—						—		—		—							

Interpretation of Surveillance Samples

Surveillance cultures allow the intensive care specialist to distinguish the normal from the abnormal carrier state, overgrowth from low level carriage, and endogenous from exogenous infections in combination with diagnostic samples.

Normal vs. Abnormal Carriage

Healthy people do not carry MRSA and AGNB, apart from the individual's own fecal *Escherichia coli* [5]. People with normal flora carry high concentrations of mainly anaerobic micro-organisms in throat and gut. There are no other AGNB, including *Klebsiella, Proteus, Morganella, Enterobacter, Citrobacter, Serratia, Acinetobacter,* and *Pseudomonas* spp., in the digestive tract besides the indigenous normal *E. coli* in the rectal swab. Abnormal carriage implies the persistent presence of MRSA and AGNB in throat and/or gut. Illness severity has been shown to be the most important factor responsible for the shift from the normal carrier status into abnormal carriage with AGNB and MRSA.

Low-Grade Carriage vs. Overgrowth

Overgrowth is defined as $\geq 3+$ or $\geq 10^5$ micro-organisms per milliliter of saliva and/or feces and is distinguished from low-grade carriage of $\leq 2+$ or $\leq 10^3$ micro-organisms. Individuals with a chronic disease such as chronic obstructive pulmonary disease carry abnormal flora once the FEV_1 (forced expiratory volume in 1 sec) is less than 50%, in general in low concentrations [6]. The low level carrier status is mainly due to the presence of clearing mechanisms such as swallowing, chewing, and peristalsis. However, long-stay patients in general have impaired motility and readily develop overgrowth [7]. Most of them receive potent systemic antimicrobials that are active against the indigenous flora of the patient, after excretion via saliva, bile, and mucus into the digestive tract [8]. Normal flora is indispensable to control abnormal AGNB and MRSA [9]. One of the consequences of using ever more potent antimicrobials, that disregard ecology, is the promotion of overgrowth of abnormal flora.

Overgrowth is a harmful event in the individual. Small intestinal overgrowth of abnormal flora has been shown to induce and maintain a systemic immunoparalysis [10-12]. Absorbed gut endotoxin is thought to play a role in the systemic immunological disorders via a systemic tumor necrosis factor (TNF) response and subsequent downregulation of the macrophages. In addition, overgrowth has been shown to be an independent risk factor for:
1. Colonization/infection of internal organs. For example, when the throat shows 3+ of *P. aeruginosa*, the chance that identical *P. aeruginosa* is in the lower airways is 50% [13].
2. Transmission of abnormal (often resistant) micro-organisms. The higher the oropharyngeal and/or rectal concentrations of AGNB and MRSA, the higher the chance of transmission via the hands of carers [14-16].
3. Expression of a resistant mutant among the microbial population. Gut over-

growth is required for the presence of a mutant micro-organism that is resistant to the systemic antibiotic excreted via bile and mucus into the gut. The fecal antibiotic levels are in general fluctuating and nonlethal and create ideal circumstances for selection of a resistant mutant, in particular in the absence of leukocytes in the intestinal lumen. The gut being the prime body site for the emergence of a resistant mutant has been clearly demonstrated for *Enterobacter* species following systemic cephalosporin administration [17].

Interaction between Carriage and Infection

With the structured approach, which combines data from surveillance and diagnostic samples (Tabs. 1, 2), infection can be categorized into three different groups [4]:

1. Primary endogenous infections are the most frequent; they are caused by both "community" and "hospital" micro-organisms carried in the throat and gut on admission. These episodes generally occur early during the ICU stay. Examples include lower airway infection in a previously healthy individual caused by *Streptococcus pneumoniae* [5], or "hospital" type organisms such as *Klebsiella pneumoniae* in patients with underlying disease [6]. The incidence of primary endogenous infection will be reduced by prophylactic parenteral antibiotics, e.g., cefotaxime, given immediately on admission, for 4 days [3,18].

2. Secondary endogenous infections are caused by ICU-associated micro-organisms appearing late in the ICU stay, in general after 1 week. These ICU microorganisms are acquired first in the oropharynx, followed by the stomach and gut. One third of ICU infections are secondary endogenous infections. Significantly, in antibiotic-free patients on admission, almost all such infections develop only in patients who have previously had a primary endogenous infection, i.e., a subset of critically ill patients who develop more than one infection during their ICU stay. Only the topical application of nonabsorbable antimicrobials as part of SDD (see below) has been shown to control secondary endogenous infection [3].

3. Exogenous infections are less common (approximately 15%) but may occur throughout the patient's ICU stay and are caused by "hospital" bacteria, in particular *Acinetobacter* spp., *Pseudomonas* spp., and MRSA without previous carriage. Typical examples are lower airway infections caused by *Acinetobacter* spp. after the use of contaminated ventilation equipment, cystitis with *Pseudomonas* spp. from urinometers, and tracheobronchitis due to MRSA in patients with a tracheostoma. A high level of hygiene is required to control exogenous infections [3].

Study Design, Patients and Methods

Enrollment

From March 1, 1999, to November 30, 1999, all patients requiring minimally 4 days of intensive care including mechanical ventilation were enrolled in this prospective observational cohort study. We documented each patient's age, sex, admission diagnosis, location before admission to the ICU, and score on the pediatric index of mortality (PIM), with higher scores indicating higher risk of dying. Oropharyngeal and rectal swabs were taken on admission, then twice weekly. Cefotaxime was administered immediately on admission, for 4 days. Oral PTA was started when abnormal flora was isolated. Oral vancomycin was added for MRSA. Topical antimicrobials were given throughout the ICU stay. The full four components of systemic and topical antibiotics, surveillance samples, and hygiene is termed selective decontamination of the digestive tract or SDD [3].

Infection

Infection was defined as a microbiologically proven ($\geq$3+ or 10^5/ml) clinical diagnosis of inflammation, either local ($\geq$++, or $\geq$100 x 10^6/l) or generalized ($\geq$10,000/mm^3 or $\leq$3,000/mm^3). All infections were classified into endogenous (primary or secondary) and exogenous infections based on the carrier status. These data were compared with the traditional categorization, using the 48-h time cut-off.

Carriage

1. The *normal carrier* state. A patient with normal flora is defined as an individual who does not carry AGNB and/or MRSA in throat and rectum, apart from the individual's own indigenous *E. coli* in the rectum.
2. The *abnormal carrier* state was defined as the isolation of one or more of the opportunistic AGNB and/or MRSA in throat and rectum, in any concentration. Oropharyngeal *E. coli* in a concentration of $\geq$3+ is considered to be abnormal.

Antibiotic Usage

The antibiotic policy consisted of older (pre-1980s) antimicrobial agents that respect ecology. Prophylaxis in cardiac and general surgery included three doses of perioperative teicoplanin/netilmicin, and cefotaxime/metronidazole, respectively. Blind therapy was based on cefotaxime and/or gentamicin for 5 days. Children showing oropharyngeal and/or intestinal overgrowth of AGNB, yeasts and MRSA received oral nonabsorbable PTA, or nystatin, and vancomycin, respectively, throughout their stay on the pediatric intensive care unit (PICU).

Antibioic use on the PICU during the study was measured, using pharmacy records denoting the daily doses of both nonabsorbable and parenteral antibiotics. The monthly antibiotic use was compared after normalizing for the number of patient days, i.e., incidence density.

Resistance

All AGNB were tested for 16 mg/l of ceftazidime and for 8 mg/l of tobramycin while S.aureus were screened for 8 mg/l of methicillin. All AGNB and MRSA isolates obtained from both surveillance and diagnostic samples were tested.

Endpoint of the Study

The primary endpoint of the study was to test the hypothesis of the usefulness of surveillance samples in the ICU. In continuously providing the pattern of carriage in long-stay patients, surveillance samples permit:

1. The identification of the subset of patients with abnormal flora requiring oral PTA and/or vancomycin; and to monitor the efficacy and compliance of the oral non-absorbable antibiotics
2. The monitoring of the level of hygiene in the unit by accurately defining nosocomial infections due to micro-organisms associated with the ICU environment, which comprise solely of secondary endogenous and exogenous infections
3. The detection of carriers of resistant microorganisms at an early stage, allowing the administration of oral nonabsorbable antibiotics combined with isolation

Statistical Analysis

Statistical analysis was performed using SPSS software (SPSS 9, SPSS Inc, Chicago, USA), employing the Mann Whitney U test and Chi square test as appropriate. $P<0.05$ was considered significant.

Results

Patient Demographics

During the 9-month course of the study, 255 children comprising 275 separate admissions were hospitalized for $\geq$96 h on the PICU and were eligible for analysis; they accounted for approximately one third of admissions to the PICU over the study period. Median age on admission was 100 days (IQR 13-740 days). The median length of stay was 8 days (IQR 5-12 days). Thirty-eight percent of the children underwent cardiac surgery, 36% were medical admissions, and 26% were general surgical patients, including burns and trauma. Sixty-five percent of children were transferred from within the hospital, one quarter from other hospitals, and the remainder from the community. (Fig. 1). Figure 2 shows the monthly presentation of the number of PICU patient days, amounting to a total of 3254 days over the 9-month study period.

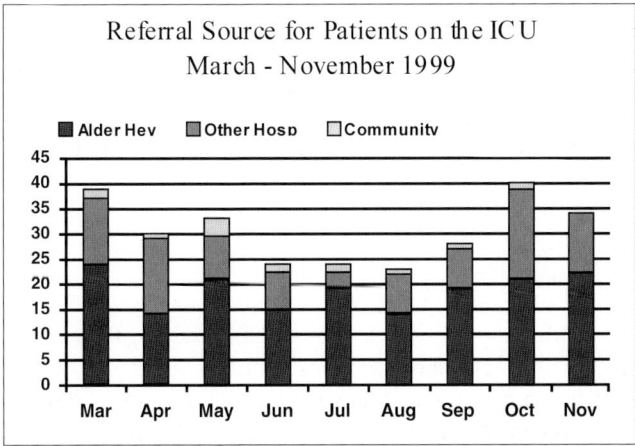

Fig. 1. Sixty-five percent of children were transferred from within the hospital, one quarter from other hospitals, and the remainder from the community

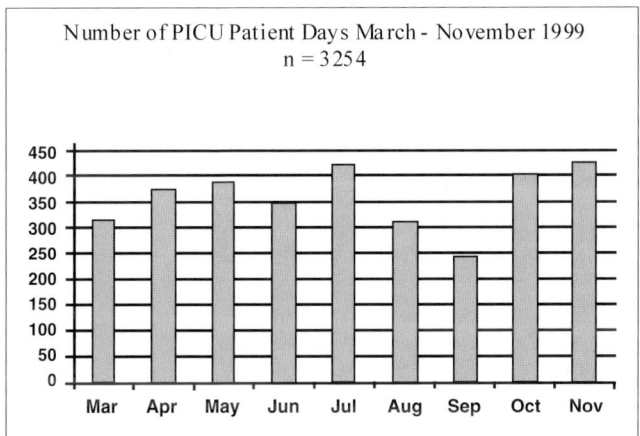

Fig. 2. The monthly presentation of the number of PICU patient days amounting to a total of 3254 days over the 9-month study period

Illness Severity Using the PIM Score

The median PIM score was 0.066, indicating that the risk of dying on the PICU was 6.6%.

Carriage

About half the patients (52%) showed normal flora on admission to the PICU. Seventy percent of the children were discharged with normal flora. One hundred

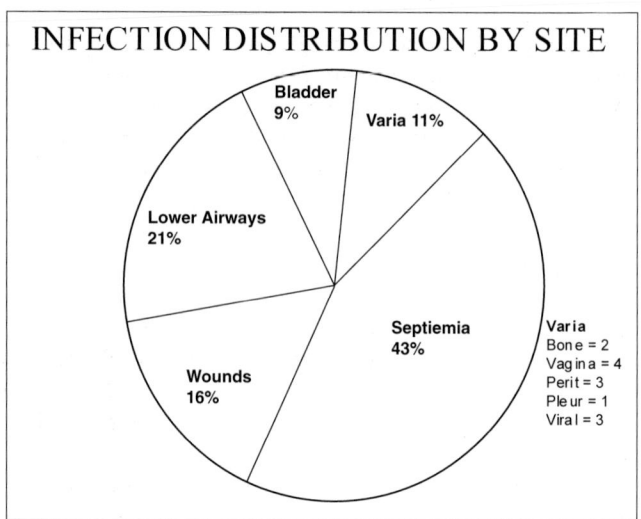

Fig. 3. Infection distribution by site detailing that blood stream infections and lower airway infections are the main infection problem in children requiring intensive care

Table 3. Microbial distribution among infections. Coagulase-negative staphylococci, *Candida albicans* and *Neisseria meningitidis* were the predominating micro-organisms causing septicemia. Lower airway infections were mainly due to *S. aureus* and RSV

Micro-organisms	Blood	Wound	Lower airway	Urinary	Varia
Neisseria meningitidis	6				
S. pneumoniae	1		2		
H. influenzae			2		
M. catarrhalis			1		
S. aureus	2	4	9		Bone
C. albicans	6	1		4	Vagina [4]; Perito [2]; Bone
Klebsiella	1	1		3	
Enterobacter	1				
Serratia	2				
Acinetobacter		1			
Pseudomonas aeruginosa	2	4	1	2	
Stenotrophomonas maltophilia	1	1			
MRSA		7	1		
Bacillus species	1				
Viridans streptococci	2				
Enterococci	3			2	Pleuritis
Staphylococci	26				
RSV			8		
CMV, parainfluenza			2		
Rotavirus					Gut
Anaerobes/aerobes					Abscess

and twenty-two children (48%) were admitted as abnormal carriers to the PICU. The surveillance swabs were still positive for abnormal AGNB and MRSA in 30% of the patients when discharged. The abnormal carriers showed a significantly higher PIM score on admission than the normal flora group ($p = 0.46$).

A total of 65 patients (23.6%) developed 121 infections with 140 micro-organisms, for an incidence of 3.7 infections per 100 patient days. Fifty-five of all infections were blood stream infections (45%), 25 lower airway infections (21%), 20 wound infections (16%), and 11 bladder infections (9%) (Fig. 3) (Table 3).

Most infections (70%) were primary endogenous, i.e., caused by micro-organisms present in the patient's admission flora (Table 4). The causative micro-organisms were coagulase-negative staphylococci, "community" micro-organisms, including *S. pneumoniae, S. aureus* and *C. albicans* and AGNB including *P. aeruginosa* and *Klebsiella*. The median onset of primary endogenous infection was 8 days (IQR 2-24 days).

The nosocomial infection rate was 8.0%, for an incidence of 1.1 nosocomial infections per 100 patient days. A total of 22 patients developed 37 nosocomial infections due to micro-organisms associated with the PICU ecology. Exogenous and secondary endogenous infections are "true" nosocomial infections as they are caused by micro-organisms not present in the patient's admission flora but acquired on the PICU. A total of 27 (22%) exogenous infections due to PICU micro-organisms not carried at all occurred in 16 patients. The predominating micro-organisms were coagulase-negative staphylococci (8 infections), *Pseudomonas* – both *aeruginosa* and non-*aeruginosa* (3 infections) – and *S. aureus*

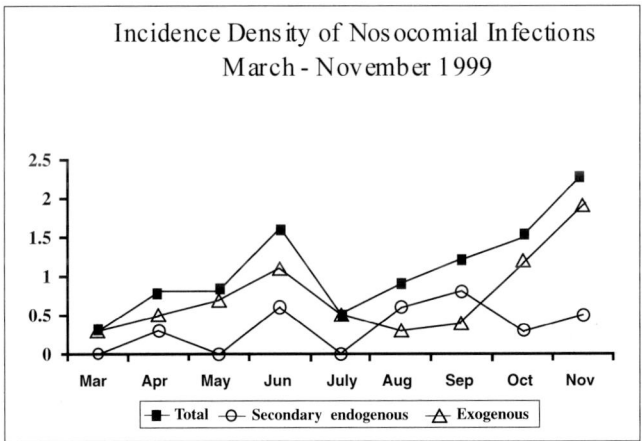

Fig. 6. Monthly presentation of 37 nosocomial infections (10 secondary endogenous and 27 exogenous infections) in 22 patients during a 9-month period from 1 March – 30 November 1999. There were no months without exogenous infections, whereas there were no secondary endogenous infections in March, May, and July always with a low incidence density of less than one secondary endogenous infection per 100 patient days. The three peaks of nosocomial infections (June, October, and November) were invariably due to a rise in exogenous infections (4, 5, and 8 exogenous infections)

– both methicillin-sensitive and -resistant (10 infections). There were no months without exogenous infections with three peaks of 4, 5, and 8 exogenous infections in the months of June, October, and November (Fig. 6). This type of infection occurred at a median of 9 days (IQR 5-16).

Eight patients suffered 10 (8%) secondary endogenous infections due to *P. aeruginosa* [3], *Klebsiella,* and *C. albicans* each 2 infections (Table 4). These ICU micro-organisms were acquired first in the oropharynx, followed by oropharyngeal and rectal carriage, before clinical symptoms of infection occurred. The monthly incidence density of secondary endogenous infections was always less

Table 4. Causative microorganisms of 121 infections in 65 patients

Primary endogenous infections (*n*=83)	
Neisseria meningitidis	6
S. pneumoniae	3
H. influenzae	2
M. catarrhalis	1
S. aureus	11
C. albicans	13
Klebsiella	3
Serratia	1
Pseudomonas aeruginosa	5
MRSA	1
Viridans streptococci	2
Enterococci	6
Staphylococci	18
RSV	7
CMV, rota, Parainfluenza	3
Anaerobes/aerobes	1
Secondary endogenous infections (*n*=10)	
S. aureus	1
Klebsiella	2
Serratia	1
Pseudomonas aeruginosa	3
C. albicans	2
RSV	1
Exogenous Infections (n=27)	
S. aureus	3
C. albicans	3
Enterobacter	1
Acinetobacter	1
Pseudomonas aeruginosa	1
S. maltophilia	2
MRSA	7
Bacillus species	1
Staphylococci	8

Pathogenesis of one infection was unknown.

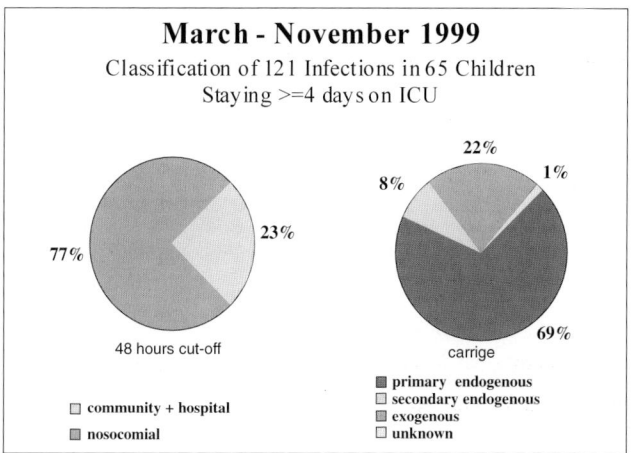

Fig. 5. Throughout the 9-month study using the concept of the carrier state, primary endogenous infections were the main problem (70%). Primary endogenous infections include all infections present on admission and all subsequent infections caused by micro-organisms present in the patient's admission flora, i.e., micro-organisms that are not acquired from the ICU environment. Exogenous and secondary endogenous infections are caused by ICU-related micro-organisms due to breaches of in hygiene. In contrast, using the traditional classification of a 48-h cut-off, there appears to be a serious nosocomial problem of 77%

than one infection per 100 patient days, while there were no secondary endogenous infections in the months of March, May, and July. The median onset was 13 days (IQR 9-105). The densities of 1.5, 1.4, and 2.5 of nosocomial infections were solely due to peaks of 4, 5, and 8 exogenous infections, as the incidence density of secondary endogenous infections was invariably low and constant.

Using the traditional 48-h cut-off, the nosocomially infected patient rate would have been twice as high with 44 patients or 16%, for an incidence density of 2.8 nosocomial infections per 100 patient days. A total of 93 infections occurred after 48 h, estimating the nosocomial problem as 77%, while the criterion of carriage detected 30% of all infections as nosocomial, 8% as secondary endogenous, and 22% as of exogenous development. This is the exact opposite (Fig. 5).

Antibiotic Usage

On average per month, 20 full days of glycopeptide therapy were dispensed per 100 patient days, i.e., a monthly density of 20% (Fig. 6). Cephalosporins and aminoglycosides were administered at a monthly density of 50% and 40%, respectively. During all but 2 months, the monthly density of topical PTA and vancomycin was higher (at 60%) than the density of the parenteral antimicrobials. Systemic antifungals were administered to only four patients over 9 months.

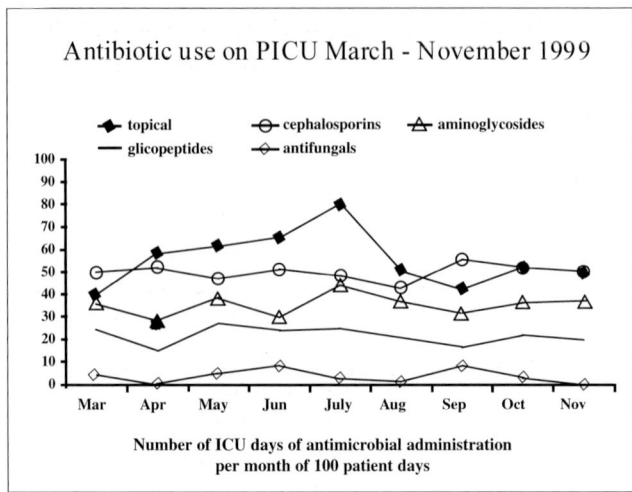

Fig. 6. Antibiotic usage. On average per month, 20 full days of glycopeptide therapy were dispensed per 100 patient days, i.e., a monthly density of 20%. Cephalosporins and amino-glycosides were administered at a monthly density of 50 and 40%, respectively. During all but 2 months, the monthly density of topical PTA and vancomycin was higher (at 60%) than the density of the parenteral antimicrobials

Resistance

Carriage

There were a total of 78 episodes of carriage of resistant bacteria in 55 patients (21.5%) over the 9-month study period. Seven patients (2.7%) were responsible for eight admissions, during which MRSA was present in their admission flora ("import"). There was no "nosocomial" MRSA. There were 52 episodes of carriage of ceftazidime-resistant AGNB in 47 patients (18.4%), *Enterobacter* and *Citrobacter* species being predominant. Eighteen episodes of carriage of tobramycin-resistant AGNB were detected in 14 PICU patients (5.4%). *Klebsiella*, *Enterobacter*, and non-*Aeruginosa pseudomonas* strains were predominant among the tobramycin-resistant isolates. Forty-eight of those resistant isolates (61.5%) were present in the admission flora. On 15 occasions (20%) patients carried AGNB sensitive to ceftazidime [12] and to tobramycin [3] in their admission flora. Following the systemic administration of cefotaxime, ceftazidime, and tobramycin, these AGNB turned out to be resistant in the subsequent samples following parenteral therapy. This conversion occurred at a median of 4 days [IQR 3-11). All AGNB were invariably sensitive to polymyxin, except *Proteus* in one patient. The carriage density varied between 1.27 and 2.71 (Fig. 7), defined as the number of patients carrying resistant micro-organisms per month of 100 patient days.

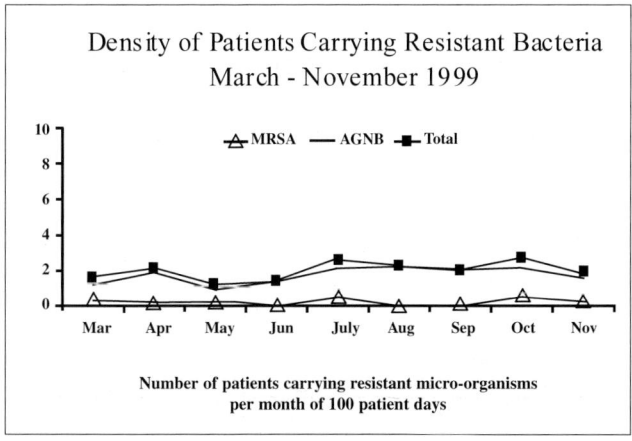

Fig. 7. Density of patients carrying resistant bacteria (March 1 – Nov 30 1999). The density is defined as the number of patients carrying resistant micro-organisms per month of 100 patient days

Infection

A total of five patients (5/255 = 2%) had eight infections due to resistant microorganisms, MRSA, *Klebsiella,* and *Enterobacter.* There were four wound infections due to MRSA (two times), *Klebsiella pneumoniae,* and *Enterobacter cloacae,* respectively: two bladder infections each by *Klebsiella pneumoniae,* one tracheobronchitis by MRSA, and one case of septicemia due to *Klebsiella pneumoniae.* All but three infections were of primary endogenous development, i.e., the patients referred from another hospital carried the multi-resistant organism in their admission flora. Two children (2/255 = 1%) developed three nosocomial infections due

Table 5. A total of five patients (2%) had eight infections due to resistant micro-organisms MRSA, *Klebsiella* and *Enterobacter* species

Patient no.	Day	Site	Pathogen	Organism	Cefta	Tobra	Gent
1	32	CVL site (groin)	Prim Endog	*Klebsiella*	S	R	
	46	Cystitis	Prim Endog	*Klebsiella*	S	R	
	63	Cystitis	Prim Endog	*Klebsiella*	S	R	
2	*8*	L arm burn wound	Exogenous	MRSA			
	8	R arm burn wound	Exogenous	MRSA			
3	3	Wound	Prim Endog	*Enterobact*	R		S
4	8	Septicemia	Sec Endog	*Klebsiella*	S	R	
5	22	Tracheobronchitis	Prim Endog	MRSA			

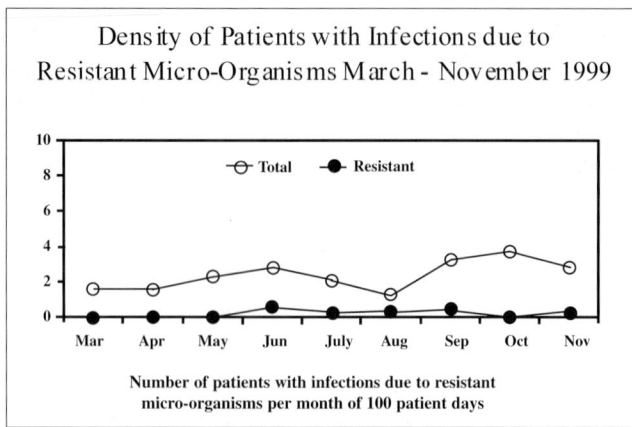

Fig. 8. Density of patients with infections due to resistant micro-organisms (March 1 –November 30, 2000). The density is defined as the number of patients infected with resistant micro-organisms per month of 100 patient days

to resistant PICU micro-organisms. One child with burns developed two wound infections caused by MRSA of exogenous development, and one child who underwent heart surgery developed a secondary endogenous septicemia with *Klebsiella pneumoniae* resistant to aminoglycosides. The median onset of these eight infections was 15 days (IQR 8-39) (Table 5). The density of children with infections due to resistant bacteria varied between 0.0 and 0.568 (Fig. 8), defined as the number of patients developing infections due to resistant micro-organisms per month of 100 patient days.

Implications for practice

The answer to the study question of whether the results of surveillance tests impact clinical management is "yes". Surveillance cultures — as part of the SDD-strategy — are indispensable in identifying abnormal carriers and in evaluating the compliance and efficacy of the subsequent administration of oral, nonabsorbable antimicrobial PTA. In addition, regular surveillance tests for the detection of abnormal (resistant) flora allowed early treatment, thereby preventing induction and spread of resistant micro-organisms. The low density of both carriers and patients infected with resistant micro-organisms throughout the study compared with traditional units supports the usefulness of surveillance cultures. Finally, surveillance cultures were found to be useful for infection control purposes, as the monthly calculation of density rates of infections due solely to ICU micro-organisms allowed the monitoring of the level of hygiene and prompt reaction in case of breaches of hygiene.

It is important to realize that, on its own, the implementation of regular surveillance samples for long-stay patients on ICU can never reduce infection. A recent

American study evaluates the impact of antibiotic restriction on the size of the endemic reservoir of ceftazidime-resistant bacteria by daily nasopharyngeal and rectal swab specimens obtained on all admissions to the ICU [19]. The message was that a ceftazidime restriction policy failed to diminish the resistance problem. However, in order to measure the impact of antibiotic policies, surveillance samples were found to be indispensable. Similarly, the interventions of handwashing [20], risk factor analysis [21], calculation of infection rates, and densities [22] have never been shown to reduce infection. Two recent meta-analyses of randomized SDD trials show significant reductions in both infectious morbidity and mortality and promote SDD to an evidence-based medical maneuver with a survival benefit of 20% and 30%, respectively [23-25].

Surveillance cultures identify a subset of patients at high risk of infection, using the criterion of abnormal carriage. One third of critically ill patients with an acute physiology, age, and chronic health (APACHE) score of 15 carried AGNB or MRSA in their admission flora [26]. Once the APACHE score increased to 27, half the population showed abnormal flora in throat and/or rectum [27]. Six studies in different populations, with trauma, neutropenia, and pancreatitis, on a medical-surgical ICU, and following heart surgery and requiring long-term parenteral nutrition all showed significantly higher infection rates in the abnormal flora group [28-33]. In the current study of patients requiring minimally 4 days of intensive care including mechanical ventilation, the abnormal carriage rate was 50% on admission. There was a correlation between PIM score and abnormal carriage. The aim of SDD is the conversion of the abnormal carrier state into normal carriage in order to resolve the associated systemic immunoparalysis [34, 35].

Awareness of carriage in long-stay patients can provide more realistic insight into the epidemiology of infection on the PICU. In our study, about 70% of infections were caused by micro-organisms carried by the patients on admission and, hence, unrelated to the ICU ecology. "True" nosocomial infections caused by PICU-associated micro-organisms included the secondary endogenous and exogenous infections. However, the pathogenesis of these two types of PICU infection is quite different.

Secondary endogenous infections are caused by PPMs that are acquired in the ICU, causing carriage and overgrowth in the digestive tract: subsequently, colonization and infection of an internal organ may occur. Aspiration of oropharyngeal secretions containing high concentrations of PPMs is the usual route of lower respiratory tract infection in ventilated patients [13]. In our study there were 10 (8%) secondary endogenous infections, with a monthly density of less than one secondary endogenous infection per 100 patient days. The low secondary endogenous infection rate is due to SDD and is in line with the results of two recent meta-analyses [23, 24].

Exogenous infections are invariably caused by ICU-associated bacteria: the PPM is introduced directly into the internal organ from the environment. Typical of exogenous infections are the *Acinetobacter* lower airway infections following the use of contaminated ventilation equipment [36] or *Pseudomonas* lower respiratory tract infection in tracheotomized patients [37]. Twenty-seven (22%) exogenous infections due to breaches of hygiene were recorded in our study. This type of infection was an ongoing problem, implying that transmission via hands is diffi-cult to prevent on a busy PICU. In a PICU employing infection prevention using SDD, exogenous infections become obvious as the secondary endogenous infec-tions remain constantly low. This explains why the three peaks of nosocomial infections in our study, the months of June, October, and November, are solely due to an increase in exogenous infections following lapses in the level of hygiene. Becoming aware of the carrier state enables the infection control team to react.

Staff cannot be blamed for primary endogenous infections, the most common infections in the PICU [38]. Surveillance cultures of throat and rectum only allow the distinction between primary endogenous and "true" nosocomial infections. The data on the carrier state both on admission and throughout PICU stay permit the monitoring of the frequency of "true" nosocomial infections. A monthly report on the densities of only nosocomial infections may be useful, as a combination of secondary endogenous and exogenous infections may highlight a transmission problem on the PICU.

The resistance data from the current study compare favorably with the tradi-tional units [39,40]. There were five patients with a total of eight infections with eight resistant micro-organisms throughout the 9-month study. We believe that the package of the four components older systemic agents, topical PTA and van-comycin, regular surveillance, and a high standard of hygiene is responsible for the control of emergence of resistant micro-organisms. Cefotaxime and gentamicin were used at a monthly density of 50 and 40 daily doses/100 patient-days, respec-tively. In contrast, the density of ciprofloxacin and meropenem was low, with 2.4 and 0.1 doses per 100 patient-days, respectively. The data on antibiotic usage sug-gest that the antibiotic policy of respect for ecology [5,8,9] in using older antibi-otics has been adhered to. The regular clinical meetings on PICU attended by a clinical pharmacist and microbiologist undoubtedly contributed to the compliance with the flora-sparing antibiotic usage. Perhaps more importantly, the monthly density of the topical PTA and vancomycin was practically always higher than the density of the parenteral antibiotic usage, i.e., the long-stay patients who required systemic antibiotics always received oral nonabsorbable antibiotics. We believe that a shift from systemic towards topical antibiotics is responsible for the virtual absence of a resistance problem. Our policy of rendering patients at high risk of overgrowth and subsequent emergence of resistant micro-organisms free from AGNB, from *S. aureus* both sensitive and resistant to methicillin, and of yeasts has contributed to the control of resistance. The fundamental difference between the traditional and SDD approach is the administration of solely parenteral antibiotics in patients with overgrowth, compared with the administration of systemic antibi-otics combined with topical antimicrobials, rendering them overgrowth free. *Enterobacter, Citrobacter,* and *Pseudomonas* species are known to harbor antibiot-ic-inducible, extended-spectrum chromosomal cephalosporinases [17,19]. Exposure to antibiotics such as cefotaxime via bile can result in derepression of the bacterial antibiotic-resistance gene and the appearance of a resistant organism, in particular in the circumstances of gut overgrowth. That development is unlikely to occur in long-stay patients who are successfully decontaminated, i.e., free from *Enterobacter, Citrobacter,* and *Pseudomonas.* Polymyxin E and tobramycin is, by design, not active against normal indigenous flora and is synergistic against abnormal AGNB, and the aim is to convert the abnormal carrier state into the normal carrier state known to guarantee virtual absence of resistance [25]. Our data are in line with previous work. The most rigorous meta-analysis summarized 33 randomized SDD trials involving 5725 patients which were conducted over a period of more than 10 years (1987-1997) [23]. There was never any emergence of resistant micro-organisms, subsequent superinfections, or epidemics of multi-resistant micro-organisms reported in any of the trials. In addition, three studies in which resistance during SDD was the endpoint fail to report resistance [41-43]. Although experts agree that surveillance samples are required to control resistance, their use is rare [44]. We believe that an intensive care specialist should be aware of what flora a patient imports into the ICU, and what type of flora the patient develops during their ICU stay. In this study, surveillance samples detected seven patients who were carriers of MRSA on admission, allowing prompt isolation and commencement of oral vancomycin treatment. All patients who imported abnormal AGNB — despite being sensitive to ceftazidime and tobramycin — received SDD, in order to prevent the emergence of resistance. It has so far been accepted that screening for carriers rather than simply identifying infected patients has a major role in the control of resistance. Finally, a high standard of hygiene is required to reduce transmission of resistant micro-organisms.

Reporting half-yearly or yearly infection rates and densities, in general, pleases chief executives and is important for publications. However, the favorable rates and densities in our unit are due to the routine implementation of SDD and not due to the calculation of infection rates and densities per se. If rates and densities are of value to infection control, they should be reported monthly so that the infection control team to react.

The Centers for Disease Control and Prevention (CDC) based in Atlanta, USA, consider device-associated site-specific infection rates as currently the most useful rates for interhospital comparisons. However, the variation in these rates between ICUs is considerable [45]. The CDC believes that a host susceptibility to infection scoring system needs to be developed to adjust nosocomial infection rates for interhospital comparison [22,46]. Our study supports previous work [37,38] showing that most nosocomial infections are not due to nosocomial or ICU-related micro-organisms. For interhospital comparison only infections due to ICU-bacteria, i.e., secondary endogenous and exogenous infections, can be evaluated, as these infections are due to breaches of hygiene only. Perhaps infection rates using the concept of the carrier state may be more meaningful for interhospital comparison [4].

References

1. van Saene HKF, Silvestri L, Baines P (1998) Definitions. In: van Saene HKF, Silvestri L, de la Cal MA (eds) Infection control in the intensive care unit. Springer-Verlag Italia, Milano, pp 1-8

2. Damjanovic V, van Saene HKF, Weindling AM et al (1994) The multiple value of surveillance cultures: an alternative view. J Hosp Infect 28:71-74

3. Baxby D, van Saene HKF, Stoutenbeek CP et al (1996) Selective decontamination of the digestive tract: 13 years on, what it is and what it is not. Intensive Care Med 22:699-706

4. van Saene HKF, Damjanovic V, Murray AE et al (1996) How to classify infections in intensive care units - the carrier state, a criterion whose time has come? J Hosp Infect 33:1-12

5. van Saene HKF, Tometzki AP, Fairclough SJ et al (1999) Carriage, colonisation and infection. In: Bion J (ed) Intensive care medicine. Fundamentals of anaesthesia and acute medicine. BMJ Books, BMA House, Tavistock Square, London, pp 272-285

6. Mobbs KJ, van Saene HKF, Sunderland D et al (1999) Oropharyngeal Gram-negative bacillary carriage in chronic obstructive pulmonary disease: relation to severity of disease. Respir Med 93:540-545

7. Donnell SC, Taylor N, van Saene HKF et al (1998) Nutritional implications of gut overgrowth and selective decontamination of the digestive tract. Proc Nutrit Soc 57:381-387

8. Eickhoff TC (1992) Antibiotics and nosocomial infections. In: Bennett JV, Brachman PS (eds) Hospital infections, 3rd edn. Little, Brown and Company, Boston, pp 245-264

9. van Saene R, Fairclough S, Petros A (1998) Broad and narrow spectrum antibiotics: a different approach. Clin Microbiol Infect 4:56-57

10. Marshall JC, Christou NV, Meakins JL (1988) Small bowel bacterial overgrowth and systemic immuno-suppression in experimental peritonitis. Surgery 104:404-411

11. Riordan SM, McIver CJ, Wakefield D et al (1999) Serum immunoglobulin and soluble IL-2 receptor levels in small intestinal overgrowth with indigenous gut flora. Dig Dis Sci 44:939-944

12. Mason CM, Dobard E, Summer WR, Nelson S (1997) Intraportal lipopolysaccharide suppresses pulmonary antibacterial defense mechanisms. J Infect Dis 176:1293-1302

13. van Uffelen R, van Saene HKF, Fidler V et al (1984) Oropharyngeal flora as a source of bacteria colonizing the lower airways in patients on artificial ventilation. Intensive Care Med 10:233-237

14. Bonten MJM, Gaillard CA, Johanson WG et al (1994) Colonization in patients receiving and not receiving topical antimicrobial prophylaxis. Am J Respir Crit Care Med 150: 1332-1340

15. Brun-Buisson C, Legrand P, Rauss A et al (1989) Intestinal decontamination for control of nosocomial multi-resistant Gram-negative bacilli. Ann Intern Med 110:873-881

16. Taylor ME, Oppenheim BA (1991) Selective decontamination of the gastro-intestinal tract as an infection control measure. J Hosp Infect 17:271-278

17. Modi N, Damjanovic V, Cooke RWI (1987) Outbreak of cephalosporin resistant *Enterobacter cloacae* infections in a neonatal intensive care unit. Arch Dis Child 62:148-151

18. Sirvent JM, Torres A, El-Ebiary M et al (1997) Protective effect of intravenously administered cefuroxime against nosocomial pneumonia in patients with structural coma. Am J Respir Crit Care Med 155:1729-1734

19. Toltzis Ph, Yamashita T, Vilt L et al (1998) Antibiotic restriction does not alter endemic colonization with resistant Gram-negative rods in a pediatric intensive care unit. Crit Care Med 26:1893-1899

20. Daschner FD, Frey P, Wolff G et al (1982) Nosocomial infections in intensive care wards: a multicenter prospective study. Intensive Care Med 8:5-9

21. Lortholary O, Fagon JY, Buu Hoi A et al (1995) Nosocomial acquisition of multi-resistant *Acinetobacter baumannii*: risk factors and prognosis. Clin Infect Dis 20:790-796

22. Gaynes RP, Culver DH, Banerjee S et al (1993) Meaningful interhospital comparison of infection rates in intensive care units. Am J Infect Control 21:43-44

A Novel Approach to Infection Control Using Selective Decontamination of the Digestive Tract

The new policy of SDD is based on three principles:

1. The criterion of microbial virulence for classifying microorganisms is preferred to the Gram stain. The target microorganisms of SDD are aerobic gram-negative bacilli (AGNB), *S. aureus*, and yeasts. Microorganisms of low virulence such as viridans streptococci, enterococci, CNS, and anaerobes are left undisturbed, as they generally do not cause death or serious infections.
2. The criterion of carriage prevails over the cut-off time of 48 h as the carrier state allows the accurate identification of the three different types of infections occurring in critically ill patients.
3. Effective SDD renders ICU patients free from AGNB. Critically ill patients who do not carry AGNB have significantly less endotoxin in their gut. A reduction in gut endotoxin is associated with significantly less endotoxin absorption and is subsequently followed by recovery of the systemic immunity.

SDD is a Four-Component Protocol

1. A parenteral antibiotic (e.g., cefotaxime, or ceftazidime if the patient is suspected to carry a pseudomonal strain) administered for the first few days to prevent primary endogenous infection.
2. Carefully selected, nonabsorbable antimicrobials such as polymyxin E, tobramycin and amphotericin B (PTA) applied topically in throat and gut throughout the stay on the ICU to prevent secondary endogenous infections; 0.5 g of paste or gel containing 2% PTA are applied on the oropharyngeal mucosa with a gloved finger four times a day; 9 ml of suspension containing 100 mg of polymyxin E, 80 mg of tobramycin and 500 mg of amphotericin B are administered in the digestive tract through a nasogastric tube four times a day.
3. A high standard of hygiene to prevent exogenous infections.
4. Surveillance samples of throat and rectum to distinguish between the three type of infections and to monitor the compliance and efficacy of the SDD.

The crucial difference between traditional methods and SDD microbiology in critically ill patients is the necessity of surveillance samples to detect the carrier state of the ICU patient [2, 3].

What are Surveillance Samples?

Surveillance samples are defined as samples from body sites where PPMs are carried, that is, the digestive tract [15]. A set of surveillance samples consists of throat and rectal swabs taken on admission to the ICU and twice weekly, thereafter (e.g., Monday and Thursday) (Tab. 1). The aim of surveillance samples is to determine the level of carriage of PPMs. Surface swabs are obtained from the skin of the axilla, groin, and umbilicus, and from the nose, eye, and ear. They are generally not

Table 1. Twelve crucial definitions

Carriage or carrier state	Is the patient's state such that the same bacterial strain is isolated from at least two surveillance samples (saliva, gastric fluid, feces, throat and rectal swabs) in any concentration over a period of at least 1 week
Normal carrier state	People with normal flora carry high concentrations of mainly anaerobic microorganisms in throat and gut. There are no other aerobic gram-negative bacilli in the digestive tract apart from the individual's own fecal *E. coli*
Abnormal carrier state	Abnormal carriage implies the persistent presence in throat and/or gut of hospital aerobic gram-negative bacilli and MRSA
Overgrowth	It is defined as $\geq 10^5$ cfu/ml of saliva, gastric fluid, or gr of feces, and is nearly always present in the critically ill ICU patient with impaired gut motility
Low-grade carriage	Low-grade carriage is defined as $<10^5$ cfu/ml of saliva, gastric fluid, or gram of digestive tract secretions
Surveillance samples	Samples from body sites where potentially pathogenic microorganisms are carried, such as digestive tract, and skin lesions (tracheotomy, wounds, pressure sores). A surveillance set comprises throat and rectal swabs taken on admission and afterwards twice weekly, e.g., on Monday and Thursday. The purpose of surveillance samples is the determination of the microbiological endpoint of the level of carriage of PPMs
Surface samples	Surface samples are swabs from the skin such as axilla, groin, and umbilicus, from the nose, eye, and ear. They do not belong to a surveillance sample protocol because microorganisms cultured from the lower part of the body (groin, umbilicus) reflect fecal flora, while microorganisms present in axilla, eye, and ear (upper part of the body) belong to the oropharyngeal flora
Diagnostic samples	These are samples from internal organs that are normally sterile, such as lower airways, blood, bladder and skin lesions. The aim of diagnostic samples is clinical. They aim to microbiologically prove a diagnosis of inflammation, both generalized or local
Acquisition	The patient is considered to have acquired a microorganism if only one surveillance sample is positive for a PPM that differs from the previous and following isolates. Acquisition refers to the transient presence of a microorganism (usually in oropharynx and gut), while carriage is a persistent phenomenon
Colonization	It is defined as the presence of a microorganism in an internal organ that is normally sterile (e.g., lower airways, bladder) without an inflammatory host response. The diagnostic sample generally yields $<10^5$ cfu/ml of diagnostic sample, i.e., urine, tracheal aspirate
Infection	Infection is a microbiologically proven clinical diagnosis of inflammation. The diagnostic sample obtained from the internal organ yields $\geq 10^5$ cfu/ml of sample or is positive in case of blood, cerebrospinal, and pleural fluid
Super-carriage/ colonization/ infection	These are the three steps of the endogenous infection developing during and after antimicrobial administration. The antimicrobial usage leads to eradication of the carriage of sensitive microorganisms associated with the supercarriage of (1) microorganisms that are not covered by the antimicrobial agent(s) (e.g., *Proteus* and enterococcal carriage during and after polymyxin and late-generation cephalosporin treatment, respectively), and (2) resistant microorganisms (after selection) (e.g., *Klebsiella* and pseudomonal carriage during and after late generation cephalosporin and fluoroquinolone treatment, respectively)

useful as surveillance samples because surface samples yielding PPMs reflect the oropharyngeal and rectal carrier state.

Diagnostic samples are taken from sites that are normally sterile, such as lower airways, bladder and blood, and are obtained when clinically indicated to find a microbiological cause of the clinical signs of inflammation.

Why Surveillance Samples?

Surveillance samples of throat and rectum represent the fourth component of the "full" SDD protocol. Only surveillance samples allow the detection of the carrier state or carriage. When the same strain of a potential pathogen is isolated from at least two consecutive surveillance samples, in any concentration, over a period of at least 1 week, the ICU patient is considered to be in a carrier state [15] (Tab. 1). Samples include throat and rectal swabs. If one surveillance sample is positive for a PPM that differs from previous isolates, the patient is considered to have acquired a PPM. Thus carriage refers to the persistent presence of a microorganism in the oropharynx and gut. An acquired PPM is only transiently present in an otherwise healthy host.

These samples have multiple values in the intensive care setting [16]. They monitor the efficacy of PTA: PTA is effective only if surveillance samples are free from AGNB, *S. aureus*, and yeasts, and they allow the detection of the resistance problem at an early stage. Moreover, surveillance samples may help clinicians to assess the level of hygiene in the ICU, to identify high-risk infection patients, to outline empirical antibiotic policies, to adjust the antibiotic therapy, and to control and prevent outbreaks of infection.

In addition, two examples show the usefulness of the detection of carriage by surveillance samples:

1. *Determination of the pathogenicity or virulence of microorganisms* (Tab. 2): The ratio between the number of ICU patients infected by a microorganism and the number of patients carrying that particular microorganism in the throat and the gut is defined as the intrinsic pathogenicity index (IPI) for a specific microorganism [17]. Indigenous flora, including anaerobes and viridans streptococci, rarely cause infection, despite being carried in high concentrations. Enterococci and CNS are also carried in the oropharynx in high concentrations by a substantial percentage of ICU patients, but are unable to cause lower airway infections. Those low-level pathogens have an IPI of 0.01-0.03, while high-level pathogens, such as *Salmonellae*, have an IPI approaching 1. There are about 15 microorganisms with IPIs between 0.1-0.3, known as potentially pathogenic microorganisms. These include the six "community" microorganisms: *Streptococcus pneumoniae, Haemophilus influenzae, Staphylococcus aureus, Moraxella catarrhalis, Escherichia coli, and Candida* spp., which may be present in previously healthy individuals. The nine "hospital" bacteria include eight AGNB (e.g., *Klebsiella, Proteus, Morganella, Enterobacter, Citrobacter, Serratia, Acinetobacter,* and *Pseudomonas* spp.), and MRSA. Those bacteria are present in patients with an acute or chronic underlying disease.

Table 2. Pathogenicity of microorganisms

Microorganisms	Intrinsic pathogenicity	Flora
Indigenous flora Oropharynx: e.g., Peptostreptococci, *Veillonella* spp., *S. viridans* Gut: e.g., *Bacteroides, Clostridium* spp., enterococci Skin: e.g., *Propionibacterium acnes*, coagulase-negative staphylococci (CNS)	Low pathogenic microorganisms	Normal
Community microorganisms Oropharynx: e.g., *S. pneumoniae, H. influenzae, Moraxella catarrhalis* Gut: e.g., *E. coli* Oropharynx and gut: e.g., methicillin-sensitive *S. aureus* (MSSA), *Candida* spp.	Potentially pathogenic microorganisms (PPMs)	Normal
Hospital microorganisms e.g., *Klebsiella, Proteus, Enterobacter, Morganella, Citrobacter, Serratia, Pseudomonas, Acinetobacter* spp., methicillin-resistant *S. aureus* (MRSA)	Potentially pathogenic microorganisms (PPMs)	Abnormal
Epidemic microorganisms e.g., *S. pyogenes, Neisseria meningitidis, Salmonella* spp.	Highly pathogenic microorganisms	Abnormal

2. *Classification of infections in ICU patients* (Tab. 3): The detection of carriage allows the distinction between the three types of infection occurring in the ICU [1]. Primary endogenous infections are infections caused by both community and hospital PPMs imported into the ICU in the patient's flora upon admission. These episodes of infection generally occur during the first week of the ICU stay. The main infection problem in ventilated patients is lower airway infection occurring during the first week of stay in the ICU. *S. pneumoniae, H. influenzae,* and *S. aureus* are the etiologic agents in previously healthy individuals requiring intensive care following an acute event, such as (surgical) trauma, pancreatitis, acute hepatic failure, and burns. Abnormal hospital AGNB, such as *Klebsiella* spp. can cause primary endogenous infections in patients with prior chronic diseases such as severe chronic obstructive pulmonary disease following acute deterioration due to the underlying disease. Secondary endogenous infections are invariably caused by the eight AGNB and MRSA, appearing, in general, after 1 week in the ICU. These PPMs are acquired in the oropharynx first, and subsequently in stomach and gut. Exogenous infections are caused by hospital PPMs and may occur throughout the patient's stay in the ICU. These infections are caused by hospital PPMs, in particular *Acinetobacter* spp., *Pseudomonas* spp., and MRSA, without previous carriage. Patients receiving a tracheostomy are at high risk of exogenous lower airway infection [18].

Table 3. Classification of ICU infections

Classification based on carrier state	Definition	Microorganisms	Onset
Primary endogenous infection	Caused by PPMs carried by the patients in throat and/or gut on admission to the ICU	"Community" and "hospital"	Early (in general within 1 week)
Secondary endogenous infection	Caused by PPMs not carried by the patients in throat and/or gut on admission to the ICU. The PPM is acquired during ICU stay, causing secondary carriage, overgrowth, colonization, and infection	"Hospital"	Late (in general after 1 week)
Exogenous infection	The causative PPM is introduced directly into the sterile internal organ without previous carriage	"Hospital"	Any time during ICU stay

How Surveillance of the Carrier State is Conducted

Sampling

Surveillance samples of throat and rectal swabs are obtained on ICU admission, and, subsequently, twice weekly (e.g., Monday and Thursday), in all patients expected to require a long period of mechanical ventilation, i.e. > 3 days. The oropharyngeal swab is rubbed over the tonsils or the tonsillar area. The rectal swab is gently introduced in the rectal cavity and afterwards withdrawn; a colored swab guarantees the presence of fecal material. Swabs are immediately introduced into the plastic holder with the transport medium and sent immediately to the laboratory.

Microbiological Procedures

Throat and rectal swabs are processed qualitatively and semiquantitatively to detect the level of carriage. Each swab is streaked onto three solid media, MacConkey, staphylococcal, and yeast agar, using the four-quadrant method. Subsequently, the tip of the swab is broken off into 5 ml of enrichment broth (BHI, brain-heart infusion) to detect the low-grade carrier state (Fig. 1). All plates are incubated aerobically at 37°C. The MacConkey plate is examined after one night and staphylococcal and yeast plates after two nights. In addition, if the enrichment broth is turbid after one night's incubation, it is then inoculated onto the three media. The plates are examined after 24, 48, and 72 h of incubation as follows:
- 24 h:
1. The plates are examined for AGNB, i.e. enterobacteriaceae, *Pseudomonas*, *Acinetobacter* spp., *S. aureus,* and *Candida* spp.

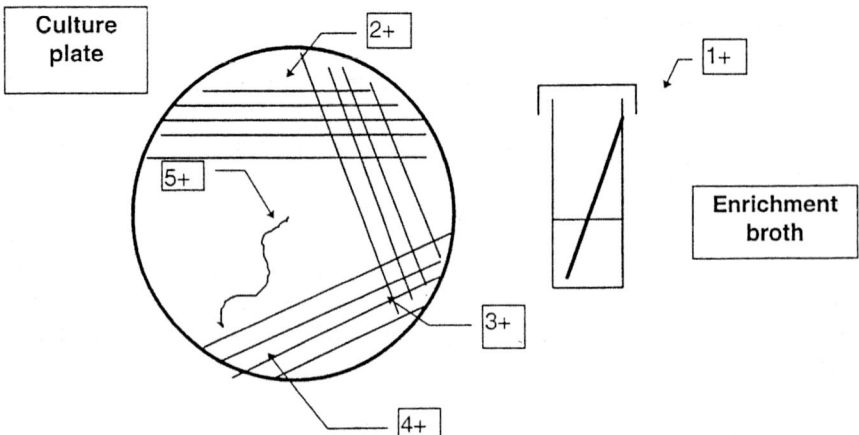

Fig. 1. Semiquantitative culture: the four-quadrant method combined with the enrichment broth

2. Staphylococcal and yeast plates are reincubated.
3. Identification and sensitivity tests are performed for enterobacteriaceae, *Pseudomonas, Acinetobacter* spp., *S. aureus*, and *Candida* spp.
4. The BHI broth is subcultured onto the same three solid media.
 – 48 h:
1. Reincubated plates and subcultures of BHI broth are examined.
2. Identification and sensitivity tests are executed as above.
3. Staphylococcal and yeast plates of the BHI broth subcultures are reincubated.
 – 72 h
1. Reincubated plates from BHI broth subcultures are examined.
2. Identification and sensitivity tests are performed as above.

Overgrowth vs. Low-Grade Carriage

The growth density is graded on a scale of 1+ to 5+ as follows [19]:

– 1+ Growth in the broth only   = Very low growth density   10 cfu/ml
– 2+ Growth in the first quadrant   = Low growth density $\geq 10^3$ cfu/ml
– 3+ Growth in the second quadrant = Moderate growth density $\geq 10^5$ cfu/ml
– 4+ Growth in the third quadrant   = High growth density $\geq 10^7$ cfu/ml
– 5+ Growth in the fourth quadrant = Very high growth density $\geq 10^9$ cfu/ml

Overgrowth is defined as an abnormally high concentration of microorganisms in throat and or gut of $\geq 3 +$, or $\geq 10^5$ cfu/ml.

Normal vs. Abnormal Flora

Normal oropharyngeal flora includes *S. viridans* in high (4+) concentrations and MSSA, *H. influenzae, S. pneumoniae,* and *Candida* spp. in low concentrations (2+) (30% carriage). Abnormal flora implies the persistent presence of *E. coli, Klebsiella, Proteus, Morganella, Enterobacter, Citrobacter, Serratia, Acinetobacter, Pseudomonas* spp., and MRSA in any concentration.

The patient's own *E. coli* is normally present in the gut in moderate (3+) concentrations. *S. aureus* and *yeasts* are carried by 30% of patients in low (2+) concentrations. Carriage of *Klebsiella, Proteus, Morganella, Enterobacter, Citrobacter, Serratia, Acinetobacter, Pseudomonas* spp., and MRSA are considered to be abnormal.

Clinical Benefits of SDD

Two recent meta-analyses have shown an important impact of SDD on morbidity and mortality (Tab. 4). The most rigorous meta-analysis examined 33 randomized trials of SDD involving 5727 patients [4]. Main outcome measures were respiratory tract infections and overall mortality. Estimates from aggregate data of 16 trials (3361 patients), in which a combination of topical and systemic antibiotics was used, indicated a significant reduction in respiratory tract infections (OR 0.35; 95% CI 0.29-0.41), and total mortality (0.80; 0.69-0.93). The analysis of 17 trials (2366 patients) which tested the effects of only topical antibiotics indicated a significant reduction in respiratory tract infections (0.56; 046-0.68) without any significant effect on mortality (1.01; 0.84-1.22). The subgroup analysis of data from individual patients did not support any difference between surgical or trauma patients and medical patients. In contrast, the hypothesis that surgical and trauma patients and patients with a high severity of the underlying disease would benefit from SDD more than other patients was confirmed by the latest meta-analysis in surgical patients compared with medical patients [20]. Rates of pneumonia were reduced in

Table 4. Main results of two published meta-analyses of randomized controlled trials of selective decontamination of the digestive tract

Author	RTIs OR (95% CI)	Mortality OR (95% CI)
D'Amico et al. (33 trials, 5727 patients) [4]		
– Topical + systemic antibiotic	0.35 (0.29-0.41)	0.80 (0.69-0.93)
– Topical only	0.56 (0.46-0.68)	1.01 (0.84-1.22)
Nathens et al. (11 trials, n. of patients not well defined) [20]		
– Overall	0.19 (0.15-0.26)	0.70 (0.52-0.93)
– Topical+systemic antibiotic	NA	0.60 (0.41-0.88)
– Topical only	NA	0.86 (0.51-1.45)

RTIs, respiratory tract infections; *OR,* odds ratio; *NA,* data not available

both subsets of patients, while those of bacteremia were significantly reduced in surgical patients only. This meta-analysis in surgical patients, though weak in design, showed a reduction in lower airway infection, septicemia, and mortality by 80%, 50%, and 30%, respectively. Only five patients needed to be treated with SDD to prevent one lower respiratory tract infection, and only 23 patients to prevent one death on ICU [4].

SDD and Antimicrobial Resistance

Surveillance samples of throat and rectum allow the detection of resistant microorganisms at an early stage, i.e., before infection and dissemination occurs. Remarkably, an interesting message of the BMJ meta-analysis is the virtual absence of any report on resistance [4]. None of the 33 randomized SDD trials included in that meta-analysis and conducted over a period of more than 10 years reported the emergence of resistant microorganisms, subsequent superinfections, and/or outbreaks of multiresistant strains. This experience is consistent with the data of three studies in which resistance during SDD was evaluated over long periods [21-23]. Additionally, two studies evaluating the resistance problem following the discontinuation of SDD failed to show any effect of SDD on the emergence of resistance [23, 24].

It is well established that the widespread use of antibiotics inevitably leads to the emergence of resistant PPMs. However, the fundamental difference between the conventional use of solely systemic antibiotics and SDD is the long-term, nonabsorbable PTA used in combination with short-term systemic cefotaxime. Mutant resistant strains generally emerge in the gut, following overgrowth of PPMs. The PTA regimen, including polymyxin E, eradicates AGNB, *S. aureus*, and yeasts, preventing subsequent overgrowth. Hence, it is highly likely that, in a patient who does not carry AGNB, *S. aureus*, and yeasts, emergence of resistance of microorganisms will not occur. Surveillance cultures are essential in the proper application of SDD, because the absence of PPMs resistant to SDD antibiotics determines the long-term safety of the SDD prophylaxis.

Paradoxically, SDD may be the answer to the increasing resistance problem, in particular of AGNB, due to the widespread use of only systemic antibiotics. PTA has been shown to control epidemics of multiresistant *Klebsiella* spp. [25, 26]. The eradication of carriage of multiresistant PPMs from throat and gut is highly likely the most effective approach to reduce transmission and subsequent outbreaks.

Impact of Surveillance Cultures on Workload
of the Microbiology Laboratory

The microbiology laboratory that provides a service to ICU patients receiving SDD will experience a shift, from diagnostic samples to surveillance samples. Fewer diagnostic samples are received due to the dramatic reduction of infection; however, surveillance samples from long-stay patients are constantly received. It is common practice in Italy and other countries to survey internal organs, including lower airways, bladder, and blood. The routine of obtaining lower airway secretions, urine, and blood from ICU patients on admission and twice weekly afterwards, even in the absence of clinical indication, is discontinued in an ICU where SDD is implemented. Tracheal aspirates and urine are only taken if they are turbid. If the patient is in a state of generalized inflammation (leukocytosis, leukopenia, fever, and high C-reactive protein blood levels), blood cultures are taken. Peritoneal, pleural and wound fluids are only sent to the laboratory in case of turbidity. In our hands, the ratio between surveillance and diagnostic samples is about 3:1.

The workload imposed by surveillance samples may be overwhelming for the microbiologist who is only familiar with diagnostic samples. However, in patients who receive the full four-component protocol of SDD, surveillance samples are only positive on admission and perhaps the next surveillance set may still yield PPMs. In patients who are effectively decontaminated, all surveillance samples are negative for AGNB, MSSA, and yeasts. The original SDD study in Groningen reports that only one third of surveillance samples are positive for PPMs [27]. One experienced technician is able to process the microbiological samples of ten SDD patients. This is in sharp contrast with lower airway secretions of nondecontaminated, long-stay patients from whom two or three PPMs may be isolated.

Conclusions

SDD is a novel concept requiring considerable commitment from clinicians and microbiologists. The four-component protocol of SDD consists of systemic antimicrobials combined with topical, nonabsorbable polymyxin E, tobramycin, and amphotericin B, high levels of hygiene, and surveillance cultures. The target microorganisms of SDD include AGNB, *S. aureus*, and yeasts. Microorganisms of low virulence such as viridans streptococci, enterococci, CNS, and anaerobes are left undisturbed, as generally they do not cause death or serious infections.

The crucial difference between traditional and SDD microbiology in critically ill patients is the necessity of surveillance samples to detect the carrier state of the ICU patient. The routine surveillance of the carrier state enables the intensive care specialist to be continuously aware of the organisms carried by the patient population and the import of a new bacterium with every new admission. In contrast, the traditional approach applies only to diagnostic samples to confirm a microbiological cause of inflammation.

Surveillance cultures have three main endpoints:
- To distinguish infections of exogenous pathogenesis (i.e., without previous carriage) from primary and secondary endogenous infections.
- To detect the carrier of multiresistant microorganisms on admission and throughout the ICU stay.
- To monitor the efficacy of PTA.

The implementation of the full, four-component protocol of SDD in critically ill patients requires teamwork. Nursing staff applies the SDD medication prepared by the pharmacist and obtain the surveillance samples from throat and rectum, and the microbiologist processes the surveillance samples and reports the carrier state, all under supervision of the intensive care specialist, who carefully assesses the implementation of SDD.

References

1. van Saene HKF, Damjanovic V, Murray AE, de la Cal MA (1996) How to classify infections in intensive care units - the carrier state, a criterion whose time has come? J Hosp Infect 33:1-12
2. Baxby D, van Saene HKF, Stoutenbeek CP, Zandstra DF (1996) Selective decontamination of the digestive tract: 13 years on, what it is, and what it is not. Intensive Care Med 22:699-706
3. Silvestri L, Mannucci F, van Saene HKF (2000) Selective decontamination of the digestive tract: a life saver. J Hosp Infect 45:185-190
4. D'Amico R, Pifferi S, Leonetti C et al (1998) Effectiveness of antibiotic prophylaxis in critically ill adult patients: systematic review of randomised controlled trials. BMJ 316:1275-1285
5. Brun-Bruisson C, Doyon F, Carlet J (1996) Bacteremia and severe sepsis in adults: a multicenter prospective survey on ICUs and wards of 24 hospitals. Am J Respir Crit Care Med 154:617-624
6. Spencer RC (1996) Definitions of nosocomial infections. Surveillance of nosocomial infections. Bailleres Clin Infect Dis 237-252
7. Garner JS, Favero MS (1986) CDC guidelines for the prevention and control of nosocomial infections. Guideline for handwashing and hospital environmental control, 1985. Am J Infect Control 14:110-126
8. Jarvis WR (1994) Handwashing - the Semmelweis lesson forgotten? Lancet 344:1311-1312
9. Ewig S, Torres A, El-Ebiary M et al (1999) Bacterial colonization patterns in mechanically ventilated patients with traumatic and medical head injury. Incidence, risk factors, and association with ventilator-associated pneumonia. Am J Respir Crit Care Med 159:188-198
10. Fagon J-Y, Chastre J, Domart Y et al (1989) Nosocomial pneumonia in patients receiving continuous mechanical ventilation. Am Rev Respir Dis 139:877-844
11. Rayner BL, Willcox PA (1988) Community-acquired bacteraemia: a prospective survey of 239 cases. Q J Med 69:907-919
12. Murray AE, Chambers JJ, van Saene HKF (1998) Infections in patients requiring ventilation in intensive care: application of a new classification. Clin Microbiol Infect 4:94-99
13. Silvestri L, Monti-Bragadin C, Milanese M et al (1999) Are ICU infections really nosocomial? A prospective observational cohort study in mechanically ventilated patients. J Hosp Infect 42:125-133
14. Silvestri L, Sarginson RE, Hughes J et al (2000) Most nosocomial pneumonia are not due to nosocomial bacteria in ventilated patients – Prospective evaluation of the accuracy of the 48h time cut-off using carriage as gold standard. Chest (submitted)
15. van Saene HKF, Silvestri L, Baines P (1998) Definitions. In: van Saene HKF, Silvestri L, de la Cal MA (eds) Infection control in the intensive care unit. Springer-Verlag, Milano, pp 1-8
16. Damjanovic V, van Saene HKF, Weindling AM et al (1994) The multiple value of surveillance cultures: an alternative view. J Hosp Infect 28:71-74

17. Leonard EM, van Saene HKF, Stoutenbeek CP et al (1990) An intrinsic pathogenicity index for micro-organisms causing infection in a neonatal surgical unit. Microbiol Ecol Health Dis 3:151-157
18. Morar P, Singh V, Jones AS et al (1998) Impact of tracheotomy on colonization and infection of lower airways in children requiring long-term ventilation: a prospective observational cohort study. Chest 113:77-85
19. van Saene HKF, Tometzki A, Fairclough SJ et al (1999) Carriage, colonisation and infection. In: Bion J (ed) Intensive care medicine. BMJ Books, London, pp 272-285
20. Nathens AB, Marshall JC (1999) Selective decontamination of the digestive tract in surgical patients. A systematic review of the evidence. Arch Surg 134:170-176
21. Hammond JMJ, Potgieter PD (1995) Long-term effects of selective decontamination on antimicrobial resistance. Crit Care Med 23:637-645
22. Stoutenbeek CP, van Saene HKF, Zandstra DF (1987) The effect of oral non-absorbable antibiotics on the emergence of resistant bacteria in patients in an intensive care unit. J Antimicrob Chemother 19:513-520
23. Tetteroo GWM, Wangevoort JHT, Bruining HA (1994) Bacteriology of selective decontamination: efficacy and rebound colonization. J Antimicrob Chemother 34:139-148
24. Saunders N, Hammond JMJ, Potgieter PD et al (1994) Microbiological surveillance during selective decontamination of the digestive tract (SDD). J Antimicrob Chemother 34:529-544
25. Brun-Bruisson C, Legrand P, Rauss A et al (1989) Intestinal decontamination for control of nosocomial multi-resistant Gram-negative bacilli. Ann Intern Med 110:873-881
26. Taylor ME, Oppenheim BA (1991) Selective decontamination of gastrointestinal tract as an infection control measure. J Hosp Infect 71:271-278
27. van Saene HKF, Stoutenbeek CP, Miranda DR, Zandstra DF (1983) A novel approach to infection control in the intensive care unit. Acta Anesth Belg 34:193-208

Chapter 9

The Role of Surveillance Cultures in Containing Antibiotic Resistance

P. TOLTZIS

Introduction

Hospital-wide surveillance of infectious diseases, organized and administered by the institution's infection control committee, is standard in modern medicine. Through passive and active mechanisms, such institutional surveillance is invaluable for quality assurance and for detecting epidemics in their earliest stages, when they are most amenable to intervention. However, surveillance culturing done at the local level in the intensive care unit (ICU), with the goal of controlling the spread of antibiotic-resistant organisms, is controversial, and the effectiveness of such practice depends upon many circumstances that vary from organism to organism and from unit to unit. There were three principal resistant phenotypes afflicting American and European hospitals in the late 1990s, namely, vancomycin-resistant enterococcus (VRE), methicillin-resistant *Staphylococcus aureus* (MRSA), and multiple antibiotic-resistant gram-negative bacilli. The following will review the factors that determine the effectiveness of infection control interventions, including surveillance culturing, in limiting the spread of these three resistant phenotypes.

General Principles

In retrospect, it appears that each of these three types of antibiotic resistance spread from hospital to hospital and into the community in a similar fashion. Each was first recognized in clusters of hospital epidemics in the 1960s (for MRSA) and the 1980s (for VRE and multiple antibiotic-resistant gram-negative bacilli). Before these seminal epidemics were controlled, discharged patients carried them into the community and then recirculated them back into acute care hospitals, where they were again transmitted to new patients, sometimes producing new epidemics. Initially, most organisms that were reintroduced into the hospital were derived from the original clone, but as the epidemiology matured and patients traveled from one hospital to another, multiple clones appeared within the same institution. Soon importation from outside the hospital became an important, and sometimes predominant, contributor to the prevalence of the resistant organism at any given time. Simultaneously, mini-epidemics occurred with one or several clones. As a consequence of these events, the situation present in many hospitals today is a complex and dynamic mixture in which many different clones are imported into the acute care environment and in which in-hospital patient-to-patient spread of both unique and epidemic genotypes occurs.

Surveillance and infection control are most effective during the earliest stages of this evolution and are most successful when applied to the single-clone epidemic. Outbreaks caused by genetically related isolates expressing each of these three resistant phenotypes have been eliminated by identifying colonized and infected patients through active and passive surveillance, geographically isolating them, and establishing barrier precautions for colonized subjects and sometimes for the entire affected unit. These measures are always accompanied by re-education sessions to ensure that the medical staff is versed and compliant with basic infection control practice. Additional measures that are sometimes employed include segregating medical staff as well as patients, intense decontamination of the environment, and strict antibiotic control. Epidemics differ from endemic periods in several characteristics, however. In epidemic situations, new cases are almost entirely the result of in-hospital, patient-to-patient transmission of a single clone. Additionally, infection is usually confined geographically, with significant contamination of the staff and environment. Endemic periods lack some or all of these characteristics and are much more difficult to address.

To help establish rational control measures for endemic antibiotic resistance, mathematical models have been developed that accurately predict the transmission dynamics of VRE and MRSA both within hospitals and community-wide [1, 2]. The principal factors that drive these dynamics are similar from organism to organism and from hospital to hospital, but their relative importance may vary. Consideration of these factors for each of the resistant phenotypes allows us to estimate how difficult they are to control and how likely surveillance and intervention strategies are to succeed. These factors can be listed as follows:

1. The probability that the organism will be spread from patient to health care worker (HCW). This probability, in turn, is a product of the number of HCW who have contact with the contagious patient, the density of colonization of the patient with the resistant bacteria, and the length of the patient's stay.
2. The probability that the contaminated HCW will transmit the organism to an uncolonized patient. This is a product (again) of the numbers of contacts the contaminated HCW has with each uncolonized patient, the duration that the HCW remains contaminated, and the compliance of the HCW with infection control measures.
3. The probability that the organism will be imported by new admissions from outside the unit. This is influenced by the patient mix and the relative prevalence of colonization among those admission groups.
4. The influence of antibiotic exposure in sustaining the presence of the resistant phenotype in the unit.
5. The importance of environmental contamination in transmission of the resistant phenotype.

Two other factors not involved in the transmission models but concerning the practicality of the surveillance and infection control strategies during endemic periods must also be considered, namely:

1. The cost of the active surveillance and control program.
2. The consequence of transmission of the resistant organism for the health of the uncolonized subject. For VRE and MRSA, in particular, in the context of low

endemicity, eradication is probably impossible or overwhelmingly costly, but stabilization is frequently achievable. Moreover, not all patient populations are at equal risk from these resistant phenotypes. Focused efforts of surveillance during periods of increased incidence in areas of the hospital where patients are at greatest danger are therefore most cost-worthy; otherwise, routine universal body-substance isolation should be sufficient.

Vancomycin Resistant Enterococci

Transmission Dynamics

Many of the factors driving the transmission of VRE in hospitals have been defined. VRE-positive patients are heavily colonized and remain so for long periods of time [3-5]. Resistance is conferred by a readily transmissible transposon that almost certainly passes from enterococcus to enterococcus within the densely populated gut [6]. VRE is isolated primarily in critically ill or chronically debilitated patients, so the length of stay of the typical VRE-positive subject is long, increasing the likelihood of patient-to-patient spread. Indeed, characteristically approximately 50% of VRE present during endemic periods in any given ICU at any given time are clonally related [7], indicating significant horizontal transmission. The main vector for this transmission are almost certainly the hands of caregivers [8]. However, hand contamination among healthy caregivers is transient. Even in outbreaks, surveys of HCW usually reveal few if any positive hand or rectal cultures [8].

However, patient-to-patient transmission accounts for only a fraction of the endemic VRE present in the hospital. In the United States, virtually all current reports of VRE indicate that many of the organisms present at any given time are polyclonal [3, 7, 9-12]; indeed, the converse of stating that 50% are horizontally acquired is that the other 50% are not. In some studies, the majority of VRE-positive patients are colonized at admission [7]. Many of these patients are referrals from long-term care facilities, which serve as reservoirs for the organism among recently hospitalized residents [5].

Endemic VRE is almost certainly sustained through antibiotic use. Exposure to multiple classes of antibiotics has been implicated in colonization and infection with VRE [3, 8]. The strongest association has been found with antecedent exposure to third-generation cephalosporins [7] to which all enterococci are resistant. Not surprisingly, an association has also been established with the use of vancomycin itself, particularly when given orally, as well as with antibiotics with broad anti-anaerobic bacterial activity, such as metronidazole [13, 14]. It is likely that VRE colonization and infection are also perpetuated by transmission from fomites. The organism can be isolated from multiple inanimate sites in the colonized patient's room, including sheets, bed rails, tables, and blood pressure cuffs [11, 12]. In periods of high endemicity, the organism can also be isolated from inanimate sites in rooms of noncolonized patients.

Consequent to these observations, isolation measures for VRE are extensive, requiring clean gowns, dedicated thermometers, blood pressure cuffs and other instruments, and single rooms [12, 15, 16]. The costs of controlling VRE, therefore, can be daunting. However, it should be noted that enterococcus is an organism of low intrinsic pathogenicity, and invasive enterococcal infection is a disease of the most critically ill and debilitated patients. Indeed, affected patients suffer from so many other risks that, in some studies, infection with VRE carries only slightly higher mortality than vancomycin-susceptible enterococcus [8, 13], despite the fact that the organism is resistant to all but investigational antibiotics. Its threat to most hospitalized patient populations is small.

Recommendations

The most appropriate, efficacious, and cost-effective way to survey and control endemic VRE is undefined. Routine surveillance cultures of all patients on admission and during hospitalization is not warranted in most situations, where maintaining standard body-substance isolation is sufficient. Many hospitals carefully monitor the number of VRE clinical isolates per month to detect changes over baseline incidence. Some have instituted more active surveillance; in our hospital, for example, all stool samples sent to the clinical microbiology laboratory are screened for VRE, and patients on selected high-risk wards are surveyed at regular intervals to determine cross-sectional point prevalence. Patients found positive by these methods are placed in single rooms with dedicated instruments and, as long as they are continent, are subjected to glove isolation (without gowns) for direct contact [12]. All rooms housing a VRE-positive patient are extensively disinfected after discharge [17]. When studied, these measures rarely eliminate VRE from the institution, but do appear to keep it in check [18].

More extensive surveillance is warranted only when the incidence of VRE colonization and infection is consistently above baseline values or clearly on the rise in selected areas of the hospital: extensive surveillance and infection control measures should be confined to areas of the hospital where VRE is most prevalent and dangerous, namely, the ICU, oncology unit, dialysis unit, and wards serving transplant patients and those with acquired immunodeficiency syndrome (AIDS). Perianal cultures obtained with a moistened cotton-tipped swab are the surveillance method of choice [19] and should be obtained at admission and weekly [12] on the affected ward. Samples may take 48 h to process, so application of isolation precautions to all admissions until culture results are known may be required in a rapidly deteriorating epidemic, to prevent transmission before the patient's status is defined [16]. Some additional interventions have been found to be effective in selected situations. These include the following: segregating patients and staff on a separate ward [1, 16, 20], significantly limiting third-generation cephalosporin and vancomycin use [16, 21], monitoring compliance with isolation precautions, and routinely obtaining environmental cultures after room disinfection to ensure elimination of the organism from inanimate surfaces [16]. VRE are sometimes resistant to all routinely available antibiotics; even among isolates with retained susceptibility to conventional antimicrobials, however, decontamination regimens for the individual patient have not been defined.

Methicillin-Resistant Staphylococcus Aureus

Transmission Dynamics

The factors driving the transmission of MRSA are similar to those for VRE, although there are some notable differences. The duration of patient colonization of MRSA is variable, but probably shorter than VRE, averaging 1 month [22, 23]; colonization is longer among patients with tracheotomies, drains, and skin lesions [24]. Moreover, the density of MRSA, which resides on the skin, is lower than that of the bowel-dwelling VRE [21], rendering it less contagious. As with VRE, most MRSA is transmitted through the hands of HCW, and similar to enterococcus, such hand contamination is transient. In most surveys, 2% or less of cultures obtained from HCW are positive for MRSA [22, 25], although outbreaks have rarely been traced back to a chronically colonized caregiver [26]. Although MRSA can colonize tracheotomies, airborne transmission is probably uncommon [22].

A recent metropolitan-wide survey in New York City produced an epidemiologic picture similar to VRE, where point-prevalence isolates among representative hospitals of varying sizes revealed both groups of clonally related organisms and many unique genotypes [27]. These observations support a model in which a scatter of originally focused clones of MRSA in large teaching hospitals became shuffled and mixed through the community to other area hospitals. Intravenous drug users and residents of chronic care facilities have long been recognized as out-of-hospital reservoirs of MRSA. However, in America, there is a growing recognition of MRSA as a community pathogen in patients with no previous hospitalization, drug abuse, or chronic illness [28-30]. In San Antonio, for example, MRSA was isolated within 48 h of hospital admission (indicating importation of the organism) in more than half of the MRSA-infected or colonized adults [28]. In Cleveland, 10%-20% of community-acquired *S. aureus* disease is caused by MRSA (M. Jacobs, personal communication).

The relationship between isolation of MRSA and antecedent exposure to antibiotics is debated [21, 31-35]. Most antibiotics do not penetrate the principal sites of MRSA colonization, namely, the skin and the nasopharynx, so the influence of antibiotic use on the emergence of resistant populations is difficult to reason [21]. While MRSA was first identified shortly after the introduction of methicillin, few contemporary studies demonstrate an association between MRSA colonization or infection with antecedent methicillin use. However, some investigators have implicated a variety of other agents. Indeed, the reduction in the incidence of MRSA in Denmark was coincident with a nationwide campaign to lower antibiotic utilization across the board [34]. One group has argued compellingly that the spread of MRSA was initiated and supported by low-dose cefazolin use, particularly for perioperative prophylaxis [35], but others have documented a negative association between MRSA isolation and the use of first-generation cephalosporins [33]. Unlike VRE, inanimate surfaces are not thought to play a significant role in the transmission of MRSA. In some notable circumstances, however, MRSA infections have been traced to a common source; contamination of hydrotherapy tubs in burn units can spread MRSA, for example, and infected or colonized patients should use this apparatus last, followed by thorough disinfection.

Like VRE, the infection control procedures for MRSA are extensive and therefore costly. Unlike enterococci, however, *S. aureus* is intrinsically very pathogenic and can cause severe, life-threatening disease regardless of age or underlying disease, albeit at low incidence. Most data suggest, however, that MRSA is no more pathogenic than MSSA [36].

Recommendations

As with VRE, low-level endemic MRSA is usually adequately addressed with universally applied body substance isolation precautions [37], which are sufficient to stabilize prevalence rates. Many hospitals have mechanisms (usually computerized) to alert hospital staff of the admission of a former MRSA-positive patient at the point of entry in order to allow isolation until the patient's current status can be determined. Clearly this strategy addresses only part of the problem, since some MRSA-positive patients are admitted and discharged without ever being identified. Efforts should be made to discharge known colonized patients as quickly as possible.

Passive surveillance performed by the institution's infection control service is sufficient to detect significant changes in baseline incidence. When such changes are detected, focused active surveillance with the initiation of barrier precautions is best directed toward areas of the hospital where the incidence of MRSA tends to be highest and where the consequences of infection are greatest, namely, the ICU, hemodialysis unit, wards caring for patients with significant dermatological disease (especially burns and diabetic ulcers), and trauma and orthopedic units. In these unusual circumstances, colonized patients are best detected by surveillance cultures obtained by rolling an unmoistened cotton-tipped swab in the anterior nares [22, 25]; culture of wounds and tracheas can increase the sensitivity of detection [22] but sampling of intact skin or stool does not significantly increase yield. However, a single round of surveillance cultures may detect as few as 50% of colonized patients, so surveillance may need to be performed repeatedly in rapidly evolving epidemics. The strictness of the isolation depends upon the rapidity with which the epidemic is evolving and the severity of the MRSA infection. Single rooms, gloves with good handwashing, gowns for very close contact, and dedicated instruments are routine. The existence of extensive skin lesions usually prompts gowns, gloves, and masks for all those entering the MRSA-positive subject's room, with the assumption of contamination of inanimate surfaces [22].

In the event that the above-listed control measures do not stabilize the growing incidence of MRSA, decontamination of colonized patients may be effective [23]. Such regimens usually include mupirocin ointment to the nares, chlorhexidine baths, and oral therapy with rifampin plus two or three additional antibiotics (e.g., trimethoprim/sulfamethoxasole, fusidic acid, or minocycline) over a period of 5-7 days. However, failures and relapses do occur with this regimen [22].

Antibiotic-Resistant Gram-Negative Bacilli

The transmission dynamics of antibiotic-resistant gram-negative bacilli during endemic periods are less defined than for VRE and MRSA, and no formal recommendations have been offered for their containment. It has been assumed that horizontal transmission through the hands of caregivers accounts for much of the incidence of colonization and infection from these bowel organisms. Although coliform bacteria can frequently be isolated from the hands of nurses [38], the importance of hands in transmitting antibiotic-resistant gram-negative rods among hospitalized individuals is not known. We [39, 40] and others [41, 42] have determined that many antibiotic-resistant gram-negative rods are detectable during endemic periods at the time of admission to the ICU, suggesting that a sizable portion of these organisms is imported into the unit rather than acquired once there. Indeed, most antibiotic-resistant bacilli isolated from ICU patients during nonepidemic periods are genetically discordant [43, 44]. This latter finding suggests that many of these organisms are components of the patient's endogenous flora and minimizes the importance of person-to-person spread. Although gram-negative bacilli can be readily cultured from sinks in the ICU, there is little concordance with organisms isolated from patients [45]. Taken together, these data indicate that acquisition of antibiotic-resistant gram-negative bacilli from other patients or the environment occurs infrequently during endemic periods in the ICU. Consequently, surveillance cultures and isolation procedures may make little difference. Further studies defining the mode of acquisition of resistant gram-negative rods are needed before rational recommendations regarding their control can be made.

References

1. Austin DJ, Bonten MJM, Weinstein RA et al (1999) Vancomycin-resistant enterococci in intensive-care hospital settings: transmission dynamics, persistence, and the impact of infection control programs. Proc Natl Acad Sci USA 96:6908-6913
2. Autsin DJ, Anderson RM (1999) Transmission dynamics of epidemic methicillin-resistant staphylococcus aureus and vancomycin-resistant enterococci in England and Wales. J Infect Dis 179:883-891
3. Bonten MJM, Slaughter S, Ambergen AW et al (1998) The role of "colonization pressure" in the spread of vancomycin-resistant enterococci. Arch Intern Med 158:1127-1132
4. Bonten MJM, Hayden MK, Nathan C et al (1998) Stability of vancomycin-resistant enterococcal genotypes isolated from long term-colonized patients. J Infect Dis 177:378-382
5. Trick WE, Kuehnert MJ, Quirk SB et al (1999) Regional dissemination of vancomycin-resistant enterococci resulting from interfacility transfer of colonized patients. J Infect Dis 180:391-396
6. Moellering RC (1998) Vancomycin-resistant enterococci. Clin Infect Dis 26:1196-1199
7. Ostrowsky BE, Venkataraman L, D'Agata EMC et al (1999) Vancomycin-resistant enterococci in intensive care units. Arch Intern Med 159:1467-1472
8. Shay DK, Maloney SA, Montecalvo M et al (1995) Epidemiology and mortality risk of vancomycin-resistant enterococcal bloodstream infections. J Infect Dis 172:993-1000
9. Dembry LM, Uzokwe K, Zervos MJ (1996) Control of endemic glycopeptide-resistant enterococci. Infect Control Hosp Epidemiol 17:286-292

10. Bingen EH, Denamur E, Lambert-Zechovsky N, Elion J (1991) Evidence for the genetic unrelatedness of nosocomial vancomycin-resistant Enterococcus faecium strains in a pediatric hospital. J Clin Microbiol 29:1888-1892

11. Montecalvo MA, Horowitz H, Gedris C et al (1994) Outbreak of vancomycin-, ampicillin-, and aminoglycoside-resistant Enterococcus faecium bacteremia in an adult oncology unit. Antimicrob Agents Chemother 38:1363-1367

12. Slaughter S, Hayden MK, Nathan C et al (1996) A comparison of the effect of universal use of gloves and gowns with that of glove use alone on acquisition of vancomycin-resistant enterococci in a medical intensive care unit. Ann Inter Med 125:448-456

13. Lucas GM, Lechtzin N, Puryear DW et al (1998) Vancomycin-resistant and vancomycin-susceptible enterococcal bacteremia: comparison of clinical features and outcomes. Clin Infect Dis 26:1127-1133

14. Edmond MB, Ober JF, Weinbaum DL et al (1995) Vancomycin-resistant enterococcus faecium bacteremia: risk factors for infection. Clin Infect Dis 20:1126-1133

15. The Hospital Infection Control Practices Advisory Commitee (1995) Recommendations for preventing the spread of vancomycin resistance: recommendations of the Hospital Infection Control Practices Advisory Committee (HICPAC). Am J Infect Control 23:87-94

16. Montecalvo MA, Jarvis WR, Uman J et al (1999) Infection-control measures reduce transmission of vancomycin-resistant enterocci in an endemic setting. Ann Intern Med 131:269-272

17. Anderson RL, Carr JH, Bond WW, Favero MS (1997) Susceptibility of vancomycin-resistant enterococci to environmental disinfectants. Infect Control Hosp Epidemiol 18:195-199

18. Morris JG Jr, Shay DK, Hebden JN et al (1995) Enterococci resistant to multiple antimicrobial agents, including vancomycin: establishment of endemicity in a university medical center. Ann Intern Med 123:250-259

19. Weinstein JW, Tallapragada S, Farrel P, Dembry LM (1996) Comparison of rectal and perirectal swabs for detection of colonization with vancomycin-resistant enterococci. J Clin Microbiol 34:210-212

20. Jochimsen EM, Fish L, Manning K et al (1999) Control of vancomycin-resistant enterococci at a community hospital: efficacy of patient and staff cohorting. Infect Control Hosp Epidemiol 20:106-109

21. Rice LB (1999) A silver bullet for colonization and infection with methicillin-resistant staphylococcus aureus still eludes us. Clin Infect Dis 28:1067-1070

22. Mulligan ME, Murray-Leisure KA, Ribner BS et al (1993) Methicillin-resistant Staphylococcus aureus: a consensus review of the microbiology, pathogenesis, and epidemiology with implications for prevention and management. Am J Med 94:313-328

23. Girou E, Pujade G, Legrand P et al (1998) Selective screening of carriers for control of methicillin-resistant staphylococcus aureus (MRSA) in high-risk hospital areas with a high level of endemic MRSA. Clin Infect Dis 27:543-550

24. Beaujean DJMA, Weersink AJL, Bloc HEM et al (1999) Determining risk factors for methicillin-resistant Staphylococcus aureus carriage after discharge from hospital. J Hosp Infect 42:213-218

25. Cox RA, Conquest C (1997) Strategies for the management of healthcare staff colonized with epidemic methicillin-resistant Staphylococcus aureus. J Hosp Infect 35:117-127

26. Mitsuda T, Arai K, Ibe M et al (1999) The influence of methicillin-resistant Staphylococcus aureus (MRSA) carriers in a nursery and transmission of MRSA to their households. J Hosp Infect 42:45-51

27. Roberts RB, de Lencastre A, Eisner W et al (1998) Molecular epidemiology of methicillin-resistant Staphylococcus aureus in 12 New York hospitals. J Infect Dis 178:164-171

28. Moreno F, Crisp C, Jorgenson JH, Patterson JE (1995) Methicillin-resistant Staphylococcus aureus as a community organism. Clin Infect Dis 21:1308-1312

29. Herold BC, Immergluck LC, Maranan MC et al (1998) Community-acquired methicillin-resistant Staphylococcus aureus in children with no identified predisposing risk. JAMA 279:593-598

30. Suggs AH, Maranan MC, Boyle-Vavra S, Daum RS (1999) Methicillin-resistant and borderline methicillin-resistant asymptomatic Staphylococcus aureus colonization in children without identifiable risk factors. Pediatr Infect Dis J 18:410-414

31. Landman D, Chockalingam M, Quale JM (1999) Reduction in the incidence of methicillin-resistant Staphylococcus aureus and ceftazidime-resistant Klebsiella pneumoniae following changes in a hospital antibiotic formulary. Clin Infect Dis 28:1062-1066

32. Ribner BS (1987) Endemic, multiply resistant Staphylococcus aureus in a pediatric population. Am J Dis Child 141:1183-1187

33. Crowcroft NS, Ronveaux O, Monnet DL, Mertens R (1999) Methicillin-resistant Staphylococcus aureus and antimicrobial use in Belgian hospitals. Infect Control Hosp Epidemiol 20:31-36

34. Monnet DL (1998) Methicillin-resistant Staphylococcus aureus and its relationship to antimicrobial use: possible implications for control. Infect Control Hosp Epidemiol 19:552-559

35. Schentag JJ, Hyatt JM, Carr JR et al (1998) Genesis of methicillin-resistant staphylococcus aureus (MRSA), how treatment of MRSA infections has selected for vancomycin-resistant enterococcus faecium, and the importance of antibiotic management and infection control. Clin Infect Dis 26:1204-1214

36. Hershow RC, Khayr WF, Smith NL (1992) A comparison of clinical virulence of nosocomially acquired methicillin-resistant and methicillin-sensitive Staphylococcus aureus infections in a university hospital. Infect Control Hosp Epidemiol 13:587-593

37. Humphreys H, Duckworth G (1997) Methicillin-resistant staphylococcus aureus (MRSA) a re-appraisal of control measures in the light of changing circumstances. J Hosp Infect 36:167-170

38. Sanderson PJ, Weissler S (1992) Recovery of coliforms from the hands of nurses and patients: activities leading to contamination. J Hosp Infect 21:85-93.

39. Toltzis P, Yamashita T, Vilt L, Blumer JL (1997) Colonization with antibiotic-resistant gram-negative organisms in a pediatric intensive care unit. Crit Care Med 25:538-544

40. Toltzis P, Hoyen C, Spinner-Block S et al (1999) Factors that predict preexisting colonization with antibiotic-resistant gram-negative bacilli in patients admitted to a pediatric intensive care unit. Pediatrics 103:719-723

41. Schwartz SN, Dowling JN, Benkovic C et al (1978) Sources of gram-negative bacilli colonizing the tracheae of intubated patients. J Infect Dis 138:227-231

42. D'Agata EMC, Venkataraman L, DeGirolami P et al (1999) Colonization with broad-spectrum cephalosporin-resistant gram-negative bacilli in intensive care units during a nonoutbreak period: prevalence, risk factors, and rate of infection. Crit Care Med 27:1090-1095

43. Bingen E, Denamur E, Lambert-Zechovsky N et al (1992) Rapid genotyping shows the absence of cross-contamination in enterobacter cloacae nosocomial infections. J Hosp Infect 21:95-101

44. Chetchotisakd P, Phelps CL, Hartsein AI (1994) Assessment of bacterial cross-transmission as a cause of infections in patients in intensive care units. Clin Infect Dis 18:929-937

45. Levin MH, Olson B, Nathan C et al (1984) Pseudomonas in the sinks in an intensive care unit relation to patients. J Clin Pathol 37:424-427

Chapter 10

Multi-Resistant Gram-Negative Bacilli: Impact of Antibiotic Restriction

P. Toltzis

Introduction

Infections with gram-negative bacilli that are resistant to one or more classes of parenteral antibiotics have become increasingly common over the past decade [1]. These bacteria express resistance to the broad-spectrum b-lactam agents, amino-glycosides, or quinolones through different molecular mechanisms, which may coexist within the same organism. They are isolated most frequently in large teaching hospitals [2] and are commonly found in intensive care units (ICU) [3, 4]. Indeed, since broad-spectrum antibiotics are disproportionately used in the ICU, it is widely held that many of these organisms originate there. This has generated considerable interest in testing antibiotic utilization policies for hospitals in general, and the ICU in particular, designed to lower the incidence of colonization or infection with antibiotic-resistant gram-negative bacteria [5, 6]. This chapter will describe two of these policies and the data supporting their effectiveness.

Enforced Antibiotic Switches

On the surface, the simplest of these strategies is to substantially limit the use of antibiotics in the ICU. This strategy is born from the belief that populations of resistant organisms expand and flourish under antibiotic pressure. The model upon which this strategy is based posits that the patient is initially free of resistant organisms and then acquires them from the ICU environment or through horizontal transmission; these resistant bacteria subsequently find a niche created by the administration of broad-spectrum antibiotics. In the setting of an epidemic, the effectiveness of decreasing or even eliminating antibiotic use to reduce the size of the reservoir of resistant organisms is well substantiated [7, 8]. In perhaps the most striking example of this strategy, a deadly outbreak of *Klebsiella aerogenes* infections in a neurosurgical ICU in Glasgow prompted the decision to eliminate all prophylactic and therapeutic antibiotics; this strategy resulted in the disappearance of the *Klebsiella* and a dramatic decrease in the total number of infections over several months [9]. Of course, modern day practice precludes eliminating all antibiotic use in the ICU, and most modern outbreaks are addressed not by reducing antibiotic use across the board, but by substituting the antibiotic associated with the resistant phenotype with another agent. Two different hospital-wide outbreaks of ceftazidime-resistant *Klebsiella pneumoniae*, for example, were controlled by reducing ceftazidime use by 60%-80%, replacing it with imipenem in one case [10] and piperacillin/tazobactam in the other [11]. However, epidemics of resistant bacteria have features which distinguish them from periods of endemic infection. Epidemics are caused by in-hospital dissemination of clonally related or identical isolates and there is heavy contamination of the environment and caregivers' hands with the same organism. These characteristics may be important for the success of the antibiotic limitation or switch strategy.

Indeed, the link between antibiotic utilization and the incidence of gram-negative rod-resistance during endemic periods is less certain. In fact, studies that have directly tested whether antecedent antibiotic exposure during endemic periods results in the appearance of an organism resistant to the autologous antibiotic have yielded mixed results. On the one hand, the study by Chow and colleagues [12] presented compelling evidence that antecedent administration of a third-generation cephalosporin is associated with the appearance of autologously resistant *Enterobacter* infection. The emergence of resistant *Enterobacter* occurred in six of 31 patients treated with ceftriaxone, ceftazidime, cefotaxime, or ceftizoxime, but in only one of 89 patients treated with an aminoglycoside and in none of the 50 patients treated with other broad-spectrum β-lactam agents [12]. Jacobson and colleagues [13] similarly found that the appearance of a gram-negative organism expressing an extended-spectrum β-lactamase in hospitalized patients was associated with prior exposure to a third-generation cephalosporin. This clinical finding has in vitro correlates. Selected species of bacteria (namely, *Enterobacter*, *Citrobacter*, *Serratia*, and *Pseudomonas*) harbor chromosomal sequences that encode extended-spectrum β-lactamases. Expression of these genetic sequences is normally suppressed through a controlling gene. Mutation of this controlling gene results in high-level constitutive expression of the β-lactamase, and such mutants are readily selected in the laboratory by exposure to third-generation cephalosporins [14]. However, the promotion of endemic resistance by antecedent exposure to the autologous antibiotic is not confined to the third-generation cephalosporins. The association between antecedent aminoglycoside use and the endemic appearance of an aminoglycoside-resistant organism has been demonstrated by some investigators as well [15].

Given these observations, several reports have tested whether the endemic incidence of gram-negative bacteria resistant to a particular agent can be reduced by institution- or unit-wide switching of antibiotics. This phenomenon has been studied most frequently with the aminoglycosides, specifically in cases where gentamicin was replaced by amikacin [16-18]. At a Veterans Administration hospital in Minneapolis, for example, the institution-wide substitution of amikacin for gentamicin resulted in a decrease of gentamicin resistance among clinical isolates from 12.0% to 6.4% [17, 18]. Reintroduction of gentamicin 4 years later resulted in an increase in the isolation of gentamicin-resistant bacteria again [18]. Kollef and associates [19] similarly enforced a deliberate switch of empiric gram-negative bacteria coverage from ceftazidime to ciprofloxacin in postoperative cardiac surgery patients. After the switch, the incidence of ventilator-associated pneumonia was reduced, almost exclusively as a result of a reduction in infections due to ceftazidime-resistant organisms. The incidence of nosocomial bloodstream infections also was reduced, but not as dramatically.

In contrast to these findings, other investigators have been unable to find a significant association between antecedent antibiotic use and the subsequent colonization or infection with a resistant gram-negative bacillus [20-23]. Hospitalized infants treated with antibiotics for a variety of reasons were surveyed by stool culture for the presence of bacteria resistant to cefotaxime, ceftriaxone, or ceftazidime [21]. Although 26 of 65 infants were colonized with a gram-negative organism resistant to these antibiotics prior to hospital discharge, there was no association between this phenomenon and prior therapy with a third-generation cephalosporin. Similarly, Carmelli and Samore tested the association between colonization or infection with *Stenotrophomonas maltophilia* and prior exposure to imipenem (to which the organism is uniformly resistant) and ceftazidime (to which most of their isolates were susceptible) [22]. Again, no association could be demonstrated.

We likewise sought to identify risk factors for colonization with a gram-negative bacillus resistant to either tobramycin or ceftazidime in a pediatric ICU [23]. Consecutive patients admitted to our unit for longer than 24 h were surveyed for resistant organisms through routine daily rectal and nasopharyngeal cultures. Over 20% of patients were found to be colonized with a tobramycin- and/or ceftazidime-resistant organism prior to ICU discharge. Colonization was associated with young age and high Pediatric Risk of Mortality (PRISM) score, but no independent association could be established between isolation of a resistant organism and antecedent exposure to the autologous antibiotic. We subsequently initiated a study to directly test whether an enforced antibiotic switch could reduce the incidence of colonization with an organism resistant to the autologous antibiotic [24]. Ceftazidime, the principal broad-spectrum β-lactam used in our unit for empiric gram-negative bacteria therapy, was prohibited unless required based on the susceptibility pattern of the infecting isolate; most use was substituted with piperacillin/tazobactam. As before, the size of the reservoir of ceftazidime-resistant gram-negative bacteria was determined by daily rectal and nasopharyngeal sampling. Despite a 96% reduction in ceftazidime use over a 12-month period, the incidence of colonization with a ceftazidime-resistant organism actually increased during the period of piperacillin/tazobactam use [24].

The differences detected in the effectiveness of antibiotic switching among these several studies may be related to two factors. The first is that the bacteria encountered in some hospitals or ICU may be coresistant to several major classes of broad-spectrum antibiotics [25, 26]. Indeed, some investigators have documented that clonally related species of gram-negative bacteria gain and loose resistance factors over time as they spread from hospital to hospital [25]. Obviously, switching from one class of antibiotics to another will have no effect if there is a substantial reservoir of organisms resistant to both. Second, there are some units in which a significant proportion of patients found harboring an antibiotic-resistant gram-negative bacillus were colonized prior to admission. D'Agata and colleagues recently documented that 18% of patients admitted to two surgical ICU in Boston were colonized with a ceftazidime-resistant gram-negative rod on admission [27].

Similarly, we found that over half of the patients colonized with a tobramycin- or ceftazidime-resistant gram-negative bacillus in our unit were detected within the first 3 days of pediatric ICU stay [28], suggesting that they had imported the organism into the unit. In both of these studies, prior, and sometimes distant, exposure to intravenous antibiotics was documented [27, 28]. In our study, however, many colonized children were residents of chronic care facilities, and many of these had never received parenteral antibiotics; others had lived at home but had had contact with an acutely or chronically ill adult [28]. Both observations suggest horizontal acquisition of these organisms outside the hospital, which would not be influenced by in-hospital antibiotic utilization policies.

Taken together, these findings indicate that, in any given hospital or unit, a proportion of patients may acquire an antibiotic-resistant gram-negative bacterium under antibiotic pressure during their acute ICU stay, others may import the organism into the unit after acquiring it during a previous hospitalization, and still others may become colonized by exposure to a heavily colonized out-of-hospital environment or household contact. The success of an antibiotic switch program in a given institution may depend upon the proportion of patients acquiring the organism in these different ways. Indeed, it has recently been demonstrated that ceftazidime use may closely correlate with the incidence of ceftazidime resistance in the ICU but not on the routine wards of the same hospital [29], presumably reflecting the different mechanisms of acquisition among different patient populations.

Finally, it should be noted that the effectiveness of antibiotic switching almost certainly is self-limiting, since resistance to the new antibiotic virtually always develops over time. For example, the hope that a switch to amikacin would not be associated with autologous resistance was foiled by the appearance of a significant number of amikacin-resistant organisms at some hospitals [30]. Ultimately, even when antibiotic switching works, other strategies will have to be pursued to replace this relatively short-term fix.

Scheduled Antibiotic Rotations

An alternative strategy of antibiotic manipulation that has been suggested recommends a fixed, rotating schedule of antibiotics in a given unit or institution. This strategy has been suggested in position papers by expert consultants [31] and in recent editorials [32], but results of such a strategy have not been reported in peer-reviewed literature. The strategy is similar to antibiotic switching, except that the switches occur frequently and regularly and employ multiple agents. Theoretically, since antibiotic pressure from any single agent would be experienced for only a short period of time, significant populations resistant to that antibiotic will not have a chance to expand. It is assumed that the agents chosen for the rotation will all have broad-spectrum activity against gram-negative bacilli, but that they will be non-cross-resistant, i.e., the molecular mechanisms of resistance to each agent will be distinct from the others. One possible schedule, for example, could rotate use of an extended-spectrum β-lactam (where most resistance is the result of hydrolysis from a chromosomal or episomal-encoded β-lactamase), an aminoglycoside (where resistance is mediated by a separate class of hydrolyzing enzymes), and a quinolone (where most resistance is conferred by alteration of the topoisomerase target).

Key issues regarding the institution of antibiotic rotation remain undetermined. These include the following: (a) the number of antibiotics that need to be included in the rotation schedule for the strategy to be successful is undefined; (b) the duration of each antibiotic period (i.e., weekly, monthly, every other month, every sixth month) is similarly undefined; (c) whether antibiotic rotation will work in some environments and not in others remains unresolved; and (d) whether the rotation can be effective even with the inevitable breaks in the protocol has not been answered. Moreover, mechanistic issues regarding the establishment of a rotating schedule of antibiotics are substantial. In almost all health care environments, multiple physicians order antibiotics. A rotating schedule will require education of all involved, a consensus that permits the suspension of choice, a physician or group of physicians or pharmacists willing to regulate and monitor antibiotic prescription to ensure that it is consistent with the rotation, and a clear set of guidelines that allows alternative medications if the clinical situation requires it. In environments where there are large reservoirs of organisms coresistant to multiple broad-spectrum agents, or where there are significant numbers of patients importing resistant organisms into the environment rather than acquiring them after admission, antibiotic rotation will probably have little effect. Moreover, in hospitals or units where several classes of antibiotics for empiric coverage of gram-negative bacteria are available, random prescription practices conceivably could be just as effective.

It must be kept in mind that the principal goal of antibiotic manipulation is to lessen the emergence of antibiotic resistance in the given patient. Rotating antibiotics in an ICU or hospital once a month or once every 4-6 months may have little effect on the endogenous flora of the critically ill patient still treated for 14 days with a single agent, a period that may well be sufficient for the expansion of resistant populations [12]. Indeed, it may make greater theoretical sense to rotate therapy in a single patient rather than to rotate therapies in a single environment. Lessons may be derived from oncologists, who have rotated chemotherapies in individuals with aggressive tumors to avoid emergence of resistant populations of cancerous cells [33, 34]. For critically ill patients with *Pseudomonas* pneumonia, for example, it is conceivable that the best way to avoid resistance of endogenous flora as well as the *Pseudomonas* itself is to treat the infection with a series of antibiotics, all with non-cross-reactive mechanisms of resistance.

Finally, it must be emphasized that antibiotic resistance is ultimately fostered by antibiotic use. Currently, it is usually impossible to accurately identify which ICU patients truly require antibiotics at the onset of a potentially septic episode and which do not. Given the morbidity and mortality associated with infections in critically ill patients, therefore, empiric broad-spectrum therapies in the ICU are unavoidable. Technologies and validated care paths that allow the rapid identification of infected ICU patients, and the avoidance of antibiotic therapy in those at low risk are urgently needed. Almost certainly, the only truly effective strategy of antibiotic utilization to avoid resistance is nonutilization.

References

1. Burwen DR, Banerjee SN, Gaynes RP et al (1994) Ceftazidime resistance among selected gram-negative bacilli in the United States. J Infect Dis 170:1622-1625
2. Itokazu GS, Quinn JP, Bell-Dixon C et al (1996) Antimicrobial resistance rates among aerobic gram-negative bacilli recovered from patients in intensive care units: evaluation of a national postmarketing surveillance program. Clin Infect Dis 23:779-784
3. Archibald L, Phillips L, Monnett D et al (1997) Antimicrobial resistance in isolates from inpatients and outpatients in the United States: increasing importance of the intensive care unit. Clin Infect Dis 24:211-215
4. Gaynes R (1997) The impact of antimicrobial use on the emergence of antimicrobial-resistant bacteria in hospitals. Infecti Dis Clin of North Am 11:757-765
5. Rice LB, Toltzis P (1997) Antibiotic use and resistance in the intensive care unit. Curr Opin Crit Care 3:348-354
6. Cunha BA (1998) Antibiotic resistance. Crit Care Clin 14:309-327
7. McGowan JE (1987) Is antimicrobial resistance in hospital microorganisms related to antibiotic use? Bull NY Acad Med 63:253-268
8. Toltzis P, Blumer JL (1995) Antibiotic-resistant gram-negative bacteria in the critical care setting. Pediatr Clin North Am 42:687-702
9. Price DJE, Sleigh JD (1970) Control of infection due to Klebsiella aerogenes in a neurosurgical unit by withdrawal of all antibiotics. Lancet 2:1213-1215
10. Meyer KS, Urban C, Eagan JA et al (1993) Nosocomial outbreak of Klebsiella infection resistant to late-generation cephalosporins. Ann Intern Med 119:353-358
11. Rice LB, Eckstein EC, DeVente J, Shlaes DM (1996) Ceftazidime-resistant Klebsiella pneumoniae isolates recovered at the Cleveland Department of Veterans Affairs Medical Center. Clin Infect Dis 23:118-124
12. Chow JW, Fine MJ, Shales DM et al (1991) Enterobacter bacteremia: clinical features and emergence of antibiotic resistance during therapy. Ann Intern Med 115:585-590
13. Jacobson KL, Cohen SH, Inciardi JF (1995) The relationship between antecedent antibiotic use and resistance to extended-spectrum cephalosporins in group 1 β-lactamase-producing organisms. Clin Infect Dis 21:1107-1113
14. Medeiros AA (1997) Evolution and dissemination of β-lactamases accelerated by generations of, β-lactam antibiotics. Clin Infect Dis 24 [Suppl 1]:S19-S45
15. Jessop AB, John JF, Paul SM (1998) Risk factors associated with the acquisition of amikacin-resistant gram-negative bacilli in Central New Jersey hospitals. Infect Control Hosp Epidemiol 19:186-188
16. King JW, White MC, Todd JR, Conrad SA (1992) Alterations in the microbial flora and in the incidence of bacteremia at a university hospital after adoption of amikacin as the sole formulary aminoglycoside. Clin Infect Dis 14:908-915
17. Gerding DN, Larson TA (1985) Aminoglycoside resistance in gram-negative bacilli during increased amikacin use: comparison of experience in 14 United States hospitals with experience in the Minneapolis Veterans Administration Medical Center. Amer J Med 79 [Suppl 1A]:1-7
18. Gerding DN, Larson TA, Hughes RA et al (1991) Aminoglycoside resistance and aminoglycoside usage: ten years of experience in one hospital. Antimicrob Agents Chemother 35:1284-1290
19. Kollef MH, Vlasnik J, Sharpless L et al (1997) Scheduled change of antibiotic classes: a strategy to decrease the incidence of ventilator-associated pneumonia. Am J Respir Crit Care Med 156:1040-1048
20. Talon D, Capellier G, Boillot A, Michel-Briand Y (1995) Use of pulsed-field gel elec-

trophoresis as an epidemiologic tool during an outbreak of Pseudomonas aeruginosa lung infections in an intensive care unit. Intensive Care Med 21:996-1002

21. Berkowitz FE, Metchock B (1955) Third generation cephalosporin-resistant gram-negative bacilli in the feces of hospitalized children. Pediatr Infect Dis J 14:97-100

22. Carmeli Y, Samore MH (1997) Comparison of treatment with imipenem vs ceftazidime as a predisposing factor for nosocomial acquisition of Stenotrophomonas maltophilia: a historical cohort study. Clin Infect Dis 24:1131-1134

23. Toltzis P, Yamashita T, Vilt L, Blumer JL (1997) Colonization with antibiotic-resistant gram-negative organisms in a pediatric intensive care unit. Crit Care Med 25:538-544

24. Toltzis P, Yamashita T, Morrisy A et al (1998) Antibiotic restriction in a pediatric intensive care unit does not decrease endemic colonization with antibiotic resistant organisms. Crit Care Med 26:1893-1899.

25. Yuan M, Aucken H, Hall LMC et al (1998) Epidemiological typing of Klebsiellae with extended-spectrum β-lactamases from European intensive care units. J Antimicrob Chemother 41:527-539

26. Jarlier V, Fosse T, Philippon A (1996) Antibiotic susceptibility in aerobic gram-negative bacilli isolated in intensive care units in 39 French teaching hospitals (ICU study). Intensive Care Med 22:1057-1065

27. D'Agata EMC, Venkataraman L, DeGirolami P et al (1999) Colonization with broad-spectrum cephalosporin-resistant gram-negative bacilli in intensive care units during a nonoutbreak period: prevalence, risk factors, and rate of infection. Crit Care Med 276:1090-1095

28. Toltzis P, Hoyen C, Spinner-Block S et al (1999) Factors that predict preexisting colonization with antibiotic-resistant gram-negative bacilli in patients admitted to a pediatric intensive care unit. Pediatrics 103:719-723

29. Monnet DL, Archibald LK, Phillips L et al (1998) Antimicrobial use and resistance in eight US hospitals: complexities of analysis and modeling. Infect Control Hosp Epidemiol 19:388-394

30. Hammond JM, Potgieter PD, Forder AA, Plump H (1990) Influence of amikacin as the primary aminoglycoside on bacterial isolates in the intensive care unit. Crit Care Med 18:607-610

31. Shlaes DM, Gerding DN, John JF et al (1997) Society for Healthcare Epidemiology of America and Infectious Diseases Society of America Joint Committee on the Prevention of Antimicrobial Resistance: guidelines for the prevention of antimicrobial resistance in hospitals. Clin Infect Dis 25:584-99

32. Niederman MS (1997) Is "crop rotation" of antibiotics the solution to a "resistant" problem in the ICU? Am J Respir Crit Care Med 156:1029-1031

33. Goldie JH, Coldman AJ, Gudauskas GA (1982) Rationale for the use of alternating non-cross-resistant chemotherapy. Cancer Treat Rep 66:439-449

34. Rivera GK, Raimondi SC, Hancock ML et al (1991) Improved outcome in childhood acute lymphoblastic leukaemia with reinforced early treatment and rotational combination chemotherapy. Lancet 337:61-66

Chapter 11

Multi-Drug-Resistant Staphylococci and Enterococci

G.L. French

The Rise of Gram-Positive Bacteria

The introduction of penicillin and other early antimicrobials in the 1940s and 1950s revolutionised the treatment of gram-positive bacterial infections, especially skin and wound infections with *Staphylococcus aureus* and *Streptococcus pyogenes*, and community-acquired pneumonia due to *Streptococcus pneumoniae*. With the exception of *S. aureus*, penicillin resistance in these organisms was uncommon. Furthermore, a wide choice of agents for the treatment of gram-positive infections soon became available, including the penicillins, cephalosporins, sulphonamides, macrolides, lincosamines, tetracyclines, rifamycins and fusidic acid. Some of the agents introduced later for the treatment of gram-negative infections, such as the aminoglycosides and quinolones, also had useful gram-positive activity. With such a wide choice of treatment, antibiotic resistance in gram-positive bacteria was not a clinical problem.

Ironically, the development of surgery and modern intensive medicine produced a more compromised patient population, vulnerable to 'opportunistic' infection with the less virulent, but inherently more antibiotic-resistant, gram-negative bacteria. This change was first observed in Boston by Finland et al. [1], who showed that from 1935 to 1957 serious hospital infections with antibiotic-sensitive gram-positive pathogens were replaced by penicillin-resistant *S. aureus* and multi-resistant gram-negative organisms such as *Escherichia coli, Klebsiella* and *Proteus* spp. In later decades, successful therapies to combat these gram-negative organisms were developed, but these in turn were replaced by even more resistant, although less virulent, organisms such as *Acinetobacter, Pseudomonas* and other free-living gram-negative species. Over the next 30 years a host of new agents was introduced for the treatment of gram-negative bacteria, and by the mid-1980s, effective antimicrobial therapy was available for almost all of the clinically important gram-negative and gram-positive pathogens.

However, the gram-positive bacteria, which had been ignored for several decades, then began to emerge in new, multi-drug-resistant (MDR) forms. This was due in part to the inherently poor activity against gram-positive bacteria of some of the newer agents used for gram-negative bacteria. In addition, some gram-positive species had slowly accumulated multiple antibiotic resistance genes, rendering them resistant to a wide range of previously effective drugs. Finally, many of the infection control procedures developed during the 1970s for controlling free-living gram-negative bacteria were ineffective against endogenous gram-positive bacteria derived from patients' own mucosal and skin flora.

The particular problem organisms of MDR gram-positive hospital infection are the coagulase-negative staphylococci (CoNS), *S. aureus* and the enterococci. All three groups show increasing multiple antibiotic resistance. Some enterococci are now resistant to all available antibiotics, and the fear that such total resistance will emerge in other organisms has led to ominous warnings of the end of the antibiotic era [2, 3].

Multiply Antibiotic-Resistant Gram-Positive Infection in Intensive Care Units

A U.S. National Nosocomial Infection Survey (NNIS) carried out between 1990 and 1996 found that multi-resistant gram-positive bacteria were responsible for 39% of all hospital infections [4]. *Staphylococcus aureus* was the commonest isolate, followed by *E. coli*, CoNS and *Enterococcus* spp. CoNS were the commonest organisms isolated from blood, and enterococci the second most common from urine (after *E. coli*). Gram-positive bacteria were also frequently isolated from intensive care patients between 1986 and 1997 [5], where they were found in 50% of positive blood cultures and 39% of infected wounds. The commonest blood isolates were coagulase-negative staphylococci (34%), *S. aureus* (13%), enterococci (13%) and *Candida* spp. (6%). In Europe, a 1-day prevalence survey of infection in 1995 in over 1400 intensive care units in 17 countries found that *S. aureus* was the most frequently isolated pathogen (30%), followed by *P. aeruginosa* (29%), CoNS (19%), yeasts (17%) and enterococci (12%) [6]. In this study, approximately 60% of all *S. aureus* isolates were methicillin resistant, but this ranged from less than 1% in many Northern European countries to 80% in Southern countries such as Italy, France and Greece.

Nosocomial Multi-Drug-Resistant Gram-Positive Pathogens

Staphylococcus aureus

Although *S. aureus* was initially fully sensitive to penicillin, resistance soon developed and became widespread: by the end of the 1940s, some 60% of hospital strains were penicillin resistant. Today, some 90% of both hospital and community isolates are penicillin resistant. This common form of resistance is mediated by the production of staphylococcal penicillinase enzymes that break down the penicillin β-lactam ring, rendering the drug ineffective. This resistance is plasmid encoded and can spread from resistant to sensitive organisms by bacteriophage transduction.

In the 1950s, penicillin-resistant *S. aureus* caused serious outbreaks of hospital infection throughout the world. In the 1960s, these strains disappeared, partly because of the arrival of the penicillinase-resistant penicillins, methicillin and oxacillin, and perhaps also because of a loss of virulence or epidemicity. Methicillin resistance occurred sporadically, but was not a major problem. There then began what has been called a 'decade of complacency', when *S. aureus* was regarded as a vanquished and rather unimportant pathogen [7, 8].

Strains of methicillin-resistant *S. aureus* (MRSA) were noted soon after methicillin was introduced, but in general rarely caused clinical infection until the 1980s. Methicillin resistance is mediated by the production of a chromosomally encoded abnormal penicillin-binding protein (PBP), called PBP-2a or PBF-2', which binds poorly to methicillin and most other β-lactams. MRSA strains are therefore usually resistant to all β-lactams (i.e. all penicillins and cephalosporins), not just to methicillin. The mechanism of resistance appears to be identical in all strains of both MRSA and methicillin-resistant CoNS, the production of PBP-2a being encoded by a chromosomal gene *mecA* [9]. The *mecA* region of the chromosome allows the insertion of other antibiotic resistance genes [10], and MRSA also acquire antibiotic resistance plasmids. As a result, MRSA tend to be highly resistant and might better be called 'multiply antibiotic resistant *S. aureus*'. Many strains are now sensitive only to the glycopeptides, vancomycin and teicoplanin.

MRSA are one of the most serious problems of hospital infection worldwide [11-13], and in most countries 20%-30% of *S. aureus* isolates are now resistant to methicillin. Epidemic strains of MRSA (EMRSA) spread rapidly between patients, usually via contaminated staff hands, and can establish themselves endemically in tertiary referral hospitals and elderly care homes [14]. Although many outbreaks are with a distinct epidemic strain, it is now not uncommon to isolate several different types of MRSA from a single hospital.

Current strains of MRSA tend to be resistant to most traditional agents and the glycopeptides remain the antibiotics of last resort for serious infections [12, 15, 16]. However, there have been recent reports in Japan, the United States, France, Germany and the United Kingdom of MRSA showing intermediate resistance to vancomycin [17-21]. These strains are sometimes referred to as glycopeptide-intermediate *S. aureus* (GISA). Their clinical significance is not clear but they raise worrying questions about the future of glycopeptide therapy. Of even more concern is the possibility that high-level vancomycin resistance may pass to *S. aureus* from the enterococci (see below). This has not yet happened in nature, but the transfer has been achieved in the laboratory [22]. The emergence of untreatable glycopeptide-resistant *S. aureus* would be a calamity, since the the whole of modern surgery and intensive care is based on the control of staphylococcal sepsis.

Coagulase-Negative Staphylococci

There are many species of CoNS, of which the commonest isolated from clinical material is *Staphylococcus epidermidis*. At one time, CoNS were regarded as insignificant pathogens of humans, but they are now recognized as increasingly important causes of infection in hospitalized and compromised patients. Many of these organisms can produce an extracellular "slime" that allows them to stick to plastic prostheses and survive on foreign surfaces within a protective biofilm [23]. As a result, infections with CoNS are being seen with increasing frequency in compromised patients. These include bacteraemia (associated with intravascular catheters and vascular grafts), endocarditis (prosthetic heart valves), meningitis (ventricular shunts), peritonitis (peritoneal dialysis catheters) and infection of joint prostheses. CoNS are now common isolates from blood cultures [31], usually associated with vascular lines, especially indwelling and long-term ones such as Hickman lines [5, 24-26].

About half the strains isolated in hospitals show multiple antibiotic resistance, including resistance to methicillin (and other β-lactams), gentamicin and the quinolones. Because of this the glycopeptides vancomycin and teicoplanin are often used for therapy and prophylaxis in high-risk patients. However, low-level resistance to glycopeptides has appeared in some hospital isolates of CoNS [27]. Colonization and infection with resistant strains are more likely with prolonged hospitalization and multiple courses of antibiotic therapy, and these should be avoided when possible.

Although CoNS may cause serious infection that needs treatment with systemic antibiotics (especially in highly compromised patients or in those with prostheses), more often the 'infection' is due to simple colonization of an intravascular line and cure can be effected by its removal. Unnecessary treatment of line infections with glycopeptides should be avoided [28] in order to lower the risk of resistance occurring in more serious pathogens.

Enterococci

Enterococci are found as normal flora of the human bowel. *Enterococcus faecalis* is the most common commensal species, responsible for about 90% of enterococcal infection. *Enterococcus faecium* occurs much less frequently, but is becoming an increasingly common cause of infection, probably owing to its greater antibiotic resistance. Although enterococci have relatively low virulence and usually cause only minor urinary tract and wound infection, they can cause more serious invasive disease, especially in the compromised patient [29].

Enterococcal infections in hospitals are increasing in prevalence [30] and now cause 10%-12% of all nosocomial infection, including 10%-20% of urinary tract infections and 5%-10% of bacteraemias [4]; they are also increasingly common isolates in intensive care units [5, 6]. Most hospital infections arise from the patient's own bowel, but outbreaks of cross-infection via staff hands or environmental contamination do occur.

Enterococci, particularly *E. faecium*, are inherently more resistant to penicillin than other gram-positive bacteria, due to the low affinity of their cell wall PBP, but they are naturally sensitive to ampicillin. They have inherent low-level resistance to clindamycin, aminoglycosides and quinolones and are not killed by co-trimoxazole. They are also usually clinically resistant to cephalosporins, including newer agents such as imipenem.

In addition, enterococci readily acquire a wide range of high-level resistances. Many recent isolates of *E. faecium* produce additional low-affinity PBP and are fully resistant to penicillin and ampicillin. Traditionally, enterococci with relative resistance to ampicillin have been treated by synergistic combination with gentamicin, but this is ineffective against the increasingly common isolates exhibiting high-level aminoglycoside resistance. High-level resistance against chloramphenicol, erythromycin, clindamycin and tetracycline is also common, as is resistance to the quinolones [29]. Some strains have now also acquired plasmid-mediated, high-level glycopeptide resistance (often referred to as vancomycin-resistant enterococci or VRE) [30-33], and some isolates, usually *E. faecium*, are now resistant to all available antimicrobials. Since the first reports of glycopeptide resistance in enterococci around 1985, the prevalence of these organisms has increased alarmingly, worldwide. The U.S. NNIS survey found that from 1989 to 1997 the percentage of enterococci reported as resistant to vancomycin increased about fifty times, from 0.4% to 23% in intensive care units and from 0.3% to 15% in general words [34]. As noted above, glycopeptide resistance has been transferred in vitro from enterococci to other bacteria species, including *S. aureus* [22].

The glycopeptides are the last therapeutic resort for all clinically important multi-resistant gram-positive pathogens. The emergence of VRE with the potential to transfer resistance to other gram-positive species, is therefore particularly alarming.

Control of Hospital Infection

The first line of defence against the spread of resistant gram-positive bacteria in hospitals is the control of hospital infection. New British guidelines for the control of MRSA have recently been published [13] and the importance of handwashing as a basic measure of hospital hygiene is being re-emphasized [35]. The prudent use of vancomycin in order to reduce the likelihood of the emergence of glycopeptide resistance is detailed in a recent HICPAC publication [47].

New Antimicrobials

Vancomycin is the drug of choice for serious infection [15, 16]. While encouraging the prudent use of existing antibiotics, new agents for emerging MDR pathogens are needed. There are a number of new drugs under development for the treatment of multi-resistant gram-positive bacteria, including new glycopeptides, quinolones and ketolides. The new class of agents, the oxazolidinones of which the first is linezolid and the streptogramin combination quinopristin/dalfopristin, but the clinical role of these new agents remains to be elucidated [9, 16].

Conclusions

Multi-drug-resistant gram-positive bacteria are causing increasing problems of infection in compromised patients, especially in intensive care units and especially in catheterised patients. The further emergence of antibiotic resistance seems inevitable and there is a real danger that high-level vancomycin resistance will spread from enterococci to staphylococci. However, with the prudent use of antibiotics, improvements in infection control practices, and the advent of new antimicrobials over the next few years, we can hopefully slow down and perhaps reverse this trend and avoid potentially untreatable infections in compromised patients.

References

1. Finland M, Jones WF, Barnes MW (1959) Occurrence of serious bacterial infections since introduction of antibacterial agents. JAMA 170:2188-2197
2. Cohen ML (1992) Epidemiology of drug resistance: implications for a post-antimicrobial era. Science 257:1050-1055
3. Neu HC (1992) The crisis in antibiotic resistance. Science 257:1064-1072
4. Centers U.S. Dept. Health and Human Resources for Disease Control (1996) NNIS report: data summary from October 1986-April 1996
5. Centers U.S. Dept. Health and Human Resources for Disease Control (1997) NNIS report: data summary from October 1986-April 1997
6. Spencer RC (1996) Predominant pathogens found in the European prevalence of infection in intensive care study. Eur J Clin Microbiol Infect Dis 15:281-285
7. Shanson DC (1981) Antibiotic resistance in Staphylococcus aureus. J Hosp Infect 2:11-36
8. Shanson DC (1992) Antibiotic resistance in Staphylococcus aureus. In: Cafferkey MT (ed) Methicillin-resistant Staphylococcus aureus. Dekker, New York, pp 11-20
9. Chambers HF (1997) Methicillin resistance in staphylococci: molecular and biochemical basis and clinical implications. Clin Microbiol Rev 10:781-791
10. Berger-Bächi B (1989) Genetics of methicillin resistance in Staphylococcus aureus. J Antimicrob Chemother 23:671-680
11. Cookson B, Phillips I (1990) Methicillin-resistant staphylococci. J Appl Bacteriol [Sympos Suppl]:55S-70S
12. Mulligan ME, Murray-Leisure KA, Ribner BS et al (1993) Methicillin-resistant Staphylococcus aureus: a consensus review of the microbiology, pathogenesis and epidemiology with implications for prevention and management. Am J Med 94:313-328
13. Combined Working Party Report of the BSCA, HIS and ICNA (1998) Revised guidelines for the control of methicillin-resistant Staphylococcus aureus infection in hospitals. J Hosp Infect 39:253-290
14. Boyce JM (1991) Patterns of methicillin-resistant Staphylococcus aureus prevalence. Infect Control Hosp Epidemiol 12:79-82
15. French GL, Cheng AFB, Ling JML et al (1990) Hong Kong strains of methicillin-resistant and methicillin-sensitive Staphylococcal aureus have similar virulence. J Hosp Infect 15:117-125
16. Michel M, Gutmann L (1997) Methicillin-resistant Staphylococcus aureus and vancomycin-resistant enterococci: therapeutic realities and possibilities. Lancet 349:1901-1906
17. Hiramatsu K, Hanaki H, Ino T et al (1997) Methicillin-resistant Staphylococcus aureus clinical strain with reduced vancomycin susceptibility. J Antimicrob Chemother 40:135-136
18. Center for Disease Control (1997) Update: Staphylococcus aureus with reduced susceptibility to vancomycin - United States, 1997. MMWR 48:813-815
19. Ploy MC, Grelaude C, Martin C et al (1998) First clinical isolate of vancomycin-intermediate Staphyloccocus aureus in a French hospital. Lancet 351:1212
20. Geisel R, Schmitz F-J, Thomas L et al (1999) Emergence of heterogeneous intermediate

vancomycin resistance in Staphylococcus aureus isolates in the Düsseldorf area. J Antimicrob Chemother 43:846-848

21. Howe RA, Bowker KE, Walsh TR et al (1998) Vancomycin-resistant Staphylococcus aureus. Lancet 351:602

22. Noble WC, Virani Z, Cree RGA (1992) Co-transfer of vancomycin and other resistance genes from Enterococcus faecalis NCTC 12201 to Staphylococcus aureus. FEMS Microbiol Lett 93:195-198

23. Christensen DG, Simpson WA, Bisno AL, Beachey EH (1982) Adherence of slime-producing strains of Staphylococcus epidermidis to smooth surfaces. Infect Immun 37:318-326

24. Christensen GD, Bisno AL, Parisi JT et al (1982) Nosocomial septicemia due to multiply antibiotic-resistant Staphylococcus epidermidis. Ann Int Med 96:1-10

25. Ponce de Leon S, Wenzel RP (1984) Hospital-acquired bloodstream infections with Staphylococcus epidermidis. Review of 100 cases. Am J Med 77:639-644

26. Elliott TSJ (1988) Intravascular-device infections. J Med Microbiol 27:161-167

27. Schwalbe RS, Stapleton JT, Gilligan PH (1987) Emergence of vancomycin resistance in coagulase-negative staphylococci. New Engl J Med 316:927-931

28. HICPAC (The Hospital Infection Control Practices Advisory Committee) (1995) Recommendations for preventing the spread of vancomycin resistance. Amer J Infect Control 23:87-94

29. Murray BE (1990) The life and times of the Enterococcus. Clin Microbiol Rev 3:46-65

30. Moellering RC (1992) Emergence of enterococcus as a significant pathogen. Clin Infect Dis 14:1173-1178

31. Woodford N, Johnson AP, Morrison D, Speller DCE (1995) Current perspectives on glycopeptide resistance. Clin Microbiol Rev 8:585-615

32. Leclerq R, Courvalin P (1997) Resistance to glycopeptides in enterococci. Clin Infect Dis 24:545-556

33. French GL (1998) Enterococci and vancomycin resistance. Clinical Infection Diseases 27[Suppl 1]:75-83

34. Martone WJ (1998) Spread of vancomycin-resistant enterococci: why did it happen in the United States. Infect Control Hospital Epidemiol 19:539-545

35. Teare L, Cookson B, French G et al (1999) Hand washing. A modest measure with big effects. BMJ 318:686

Chapter 12

Therapeutic Options for the Treatment of Gram-Positive Infections

A.R. De Gaudio

Introduction

The hospital intensive care unit (ICU) has been characterized as a breeding ground for antibiotic resistance. During the last decade, intensive care specialists have had to cope with increasingly resistant gram–positive pathogens. This evolving problem is related to: (a) the high proportion of neutropenic and immunocompromised patients; (b) the use of indwelling vascular access devices, and (c) the large use of drugs with activity directed against gram-negative bacilli.

By the end of the 1950s, at least 85% of *Staphilococcus aureus* strains were resistant to penicillin. The introduction in 1959 of the new semisynthetic penicillins (methicillin and oxacillin), which are not inactivated by penicillinase, was expected to be a break in the problem of resistance. Unfortunately, methicillin-resistant *S. aureus* (MRSA) was detected in 1961 and in the last 30 years the percentage of MRSA has fluctuated in Europe from 1-2% to the alarming rate of 30-40 % in Spain, France, and Italy [1].

From 1988 until now, vancomycin-resistant enterococci (VRE) have emerged, especially in the USA where they were responsible for almost 8% of all nosocomial enterococcal infections in 1993 [2].

In 1996, the first documented clinical infection due to *S. aureus* with intermediate resistance to vancomycin was diagnosed in Japan [3] and in 1997 two infections due to *S. aureus* with reduced susceptibility to vancomycin were identified in the USA [4]. Because of the emergence of these resistant organisms, the need to find new alternatives for treatment of these infections has increased.

MRSA Infections: Present and Future Treatment

The main bacterial targets of the β-lactam antibiotics in *S. aureus* are the penicillin-binding proteins (PBPs), enzymes which have a functional role in the biosynthesis of the bacterial cell wall. The antibacterial effect of β-lactams is mediated primarily by inactivation of PBP1a and PBP1b, or PBP2 and PBP3. All the strains of *S. aureus* that are highly resistant to methicillin produce an additional PBP2a encoded by the *mec* A gene. Production of this additional PBP confers an intrinsic resistance to methicillin, oxacillin, and all β-lactams [1].

The effect of a combination of a β-lactam with a penicillinase inhibitor against MRSA has been studied. Experimental studies have shown that the affinities of both amoxicillin and penicillin G for PBP2a were more than tenfold greater than those of methicillin and oxacillin, and that amoxicillin combined with clavulanate, which protected amoxicillin from penicillinase inactivation, was at least as effective as vancomycin in the treatment of experimental MRSA endocarditis in rats [1]. Although attractive, the in vitro efficacy of this combination has not been confirmed to date by clinical trials. One of the probable limitations of the combination is that large doses of clavulanate would be required to be effective, which may not be possible in a clinical setting [1].

Because isolates of MRSA are also resistant to other antistaphylococcal agents, the treatment of MRSA infections is always limited to either vancomycin or teicoplanin. Vancomycin has a moderate extravascular diffusion and its time-dependent slow bactericidal effect may partly lower its effectiveness in vivo [5]. For this reason, continuous infusion seems necessary to obtain the best bactericidal effect [6]. In contrast, teicoplanin seems to be more efficacious and well-tolerated, offering the advantage of a single-day dose [7].

Among the new antibiotics under investigation, the potential activity of new synthetic carbapenems based on their high degree of affinity for PBP2a seems very promising. Preliminary studies in experimental endocarditis have shown that this agent was at least as effective as vancomycin against MRSA [8].

Future fluoroquinolones with a very high affinity for the mutated targets topoisomerase IV and gyrase might bypass the resistance observed toward the actual fluoroquinolone compounds [1].

Oxazolidinones, a new class of antimicrobial agents that inhibit initiation of bacterial protein synthesis have shown an interesting activity against MRSA both in vitro and in animal models [1, 9].

At the moment, the first injectable streptogramin (quinupristin-dalfopristin) represents an alternative to glycopeptides against MRSA (see below).

VRE Infections: Therapeutic Options

In VRE, some data indicated the presence of two genes that are involved in an inducible mechanism of glycopeptide resistance [10]. The phenotypes, van A and van B, which produced either high–level or low–level glycopeptide resistance, have been described mainly in *Enterococcus faecium* and *E. faecalis*. The van A is defined by an high-level resistance to vancomycin and teicoplanin, whereas the van B type is associated with variable levels of resistance to vancomycin but remains susceptible to teicoplanin [1, 10]. The van C phenotype corresponds to a resistance present in most of *E. gallinarium*, *E. casseliflavus*, and *E. flavescens* characterized by a low-level vancomycin resistance but a persistent teicoplanin susceptibility [11].

The traditional treatment of systemic enterococcal infections is based on the bactericidal combination of a cell wall-active antibiotic (β-lactam) plus an aminoglycoside. Triple combinations that associate a β-lactam with a glycopeptide and gentamicin may be effective in vitro and in animal models of endocarditis against van A strains that are resistant to amoxicillin but not to aminoglycosides, even though the synergistic effect between β-lactams and glycopeptides is still controversial [1].

New semi-synthetic glycopeptides are also an interesting option for the future.

With a still unknown mechanism of action, they have shown a tenfold to 30-fold increased activity in vitro against VRE compared with vancomycin [1]. Among the new fluoroquinolones, clinafloxacin and sparfloxacin seem to have the greatest activity against enterococci in vitro and they have shown interesting results in experimental animals [1]. Glycylcyclines, which are related to tetracyclines, have shown good activity in vitro against resistant enterococci [1].

According to Michel and Gutmann [1], a practical approach for VRE infection may be proposed in this following scheme:

1. Nonspecific preventive measures and enteric eradication with oral bacitracin.
2. If the systemic infection is due to VRE van A type, the level of resistance to amoxicillin and the combination amoxicillin plus aminoglycoside used must be considered. If the resistance is intermediate to amoxicillin, the triple association (amoxycillin, teicoplanin and aminoglycoside) could be effective.
3. If the level of resistance to amoxicillin is high, a possible triple combination is ceftriaxone plus teicoplanin and gentamicin.
4. The systemic infection due to VRE van B type must be treated with amoxicillin plus aminoglycoside or, in case of a high resistance to amoxicillin, with teicoplanin in combination with an aminoglycoside.
5. Future approaches are represented by: streptogramins (quinupristin/dalfopristin), linezolid, new glycopeptides, new fluoroquinolones (clinafloxacin, sparfloxacin) and glycylcyclines.

The Promising Alternative: Quinupristin/Dalfopristin

Quinupristin/dalfopristin (Q/D) belongs to the family of streptogramins, which represents a unique class of antibacterials in that each member of the class consists of at least two structurally unrelated molecules: group A streptogramins (macrolactones) and group B streptogramins (cyclic hexadepsipeptides) [12].

Both group A and group B streptogramins inhibit protein synthesis at the ribosomal level, and they act synergistically against many isolates, their combination generating bactericidal activities and reducing the possibility of emergence of resistant strains. The mechanisms of acquired resistance to group B streptogramins are similar to those induced by erythromycin, but group A streptogramins remain unaffected by target modifications and active efflux [12].

The pharmacokinetic parameters of group A and group B streptogramins in blood are quite similar. In addition, both the A and B groups penetrate and accumulate in macrophages and in the bacterial vegetations of experimental endocarditis. These are important structural and biological differences between the streptogramins and the macrolides. The main differentiating features are the rapid antibacterial killing of streptogramins and the rarity of cross-resistance between the two groups of antibiotics. Most gram-positive organisms are highly susceptible to the streptogramin Q/D [12].

Minimum inhibitory concentrations for 90% of isolates (MIC90) were < or = 1 mg/l for *S. aureus, S. epidermidis, S. haemolyticus, Streptococcus pneumoniae, S. pyogenes,* and *Listeria monocytogenes.*

Q/D shows similar activity against methicillin-susceptible and -resistant strains of *S. aureus*, and streptococci with benzylpenicillin (penicillin G)- or erythromycin-acquired resistance. Enterococci have a different susceptibility to Q/D, although most isolates tested are susceptible to the drug, including vancomycin-resistant and multiresistant *Enterococcus faecium*. Unfortunatly, *E. faecalis* is generally the least susceptible.

Among the gram-negative respiratory pathogens, *Moraxella catarrhalis* is susceptible and *Haemophilus influenzae* is moderately susceptible to Q/D; however, Enterobacteriaceae, *Pseudomonas aeruginosa* and *Acinetobacter* spp. are resistant. The drug is active against the anaerobic organisms tested, including *Clostridium perfringens, Lactobacillus* spp., *Bacteroides fragilis*, and *Peptostreptococcus*. Synergy has been demonstrated in vancomycin-resistant and multiresistant *E. faecium*, and methicillin-sensitive and -resistant *S. aureus* with the combination of vancomycin and Q/D.

Q/D shows antibacterial activity in vivo in animal models of infections, including methicillin-sensitive and -resistant *S. aureus* infection in rabbits, *S. aureus* and *S. pneumoniae* in mice, and erythromycin-sensitive and -resistant viridans group streptococci infections in rats [12].

The drug is rapidly bactericidal against gram-positive organisms (with the exception of enterococci and some MRSA MLSbc strains) at concentrations similar to or within four fold of the MIC, and it has a long postantibiotic effect both in vitro and in vivo.

Published data regarding the clinical efficacy of this antimicrobial agent are actually limited. The efficacy and safety of i.v. Q/D administration was evaluated in three phase 3 clinical trials: two in the treatment of skin and skin structure infections (SSSI), and one in nosocomial pneumonia (NP). Q/D was administered at 7.5 mg/kg every 8 h (in NP aztreonam was added) or every 12 h in SSSI, vs. Vancomycin (V) 1 g every 12 h (in SSSI another treatment against MSSA could be used) for > 5 day showing a favorable clinical response [13].

Skin and Skin Structure Infections

In both the studies, a total number of 893 patients were enrolled in US and European countries (worldwide study), 450 in the Q/D group and 443 in the compared group (vancomycin, cefazolin or oxacillin). The most commonly treated infections were erisipelas, traumatic wound infections, clean surgical infections, severe carbunculosis, and infection at a central venous insertion site. The most common isolated pathogens were *S. aureus and S. epidermidis*, and *Streptococcus* spp. In the worldwide study, the clinical success rate in evaluable population was 71.2% for Q/D and 72.5% for the compared group; in all the bacteriologically evaluable patients, these rates were, respectively, 71.1% and 67.1%. In the US study, the clinical success rate in the evaluable population was 64.7% for Q/D and 68.3% for the compared group.

Nocosomial Pneumonia

A total of 298 patients were enrolled in 111 centers in five countries [14]: 150 patients received Q/D and 148 received vancomycin; 171 of 198 were also bacteriologically evaluable. The clinical response rate in this population was 56.3% for Q/D and 58.3% for V. Taking into account the intubated population, the rate was respectively 54.3% for Q/D and 53.7% for V. *S. aureus* was the most commonly isolated pathogen: the eradication rate was 57.7% vs. 60%, while in evaluable patients with *S. aureus* this rate was 52.9% for Q/D and 50% for V.

The overall safety profile was similar for Q/D and the compared group (gastrointestinal events were the most common adverse events reported in phase 3 clinical trials). Venous intolerance was more frequent in the Q/D group, when administered by a peripheral i.v. route. The phase 3 studies demonstrated that the efficacy of Q/D is statistically equivalent to the control group (vancomycin, cefazolin or oxacillin) in the treatment of patients with NP or complicated SSSI.

The efficacy and safety of Q/D were also assessed in a noncomparative phase 3 study and an emergency-use study [15]. A total of 401 patients with vanconmycin-resistant *E. faecium* infection were enrolled. The enrolled patients had signs and symptoms consistent with active gram-positive infections and no existing alternative therapy: (1) pathogen resistant to all clinically appropriate antibiotics (CAA); (2) patient intolerant to CAA; and (3) documented treatment failure with all CAA. The recommended dose was 7.5 mg/kg every 8 h. This patient population had severe underlying co-morbidities, including organ transplantation, hematologic disorders, respiratory failure requiring mechanical ventilation, and dialysis. The clinical response rate (cure + improvement) was 73.8% of 193 clinically evaluable patients and 70.5% of 156 bacteriologically evaluable patients. The bacteriological response rate was 70.5% of 156 bacteriologically evaluable patients. The overall success rate was 65.4% in the treated population. The drug was generally well tolerated; the most frequently reported adverse events were venous intolerance, arthralgia, and myalgia [15].

An increase in conjugated bilirubin and interactions with drugs metabolized by the cytochrome P 450 isoenzyme 3A4 (e.g., midazolam) were reported [16]. These side effects were generally mild and transient and disappeared when the agent was discontinued.

In the case of compassionate use [15], Q/D therapy led to a very favorable success rate, despite the critical conditions of the patients and the fact that the available antibiotics were not able to cure the infections caused by multiresistant gram-postive pathogens (VREF).

At this moment, Q/D can be considered a valid therapeutic alternative to glycopeptides, especially in severely ill patients affected by multiresistant gram-positive pathogens and/or in patients with renal failure [16].

Conclusions

The emergence of multiple drug resistance among S. *aureus* and enterococci is a serious public health issue. This problem is also increasing in the intensive care setting where gram-positive bacteria are the most common nosocomial pathogens.

During the past few years much effort has been devoted to limiting the spread of MRSA and to understanding the mechanisms of methicillin resistance in S. *aureus* and the mechanisms of glycopeptide resistance in both S. *aureus* and enterococci. The transfer of enterococcal glycopeptide resistance to S. *aureus* is a major problem because it has been demonstrated in vitro that van A and van B determinants are extremely mobile [1].

While no one can predict when MRSA will choose to acquire high-level resistance to glycopeptides, a strict enforcement of preventive measures, restricted use of glycopeptides, and the development of alternative antimicrobial strategies represent the best response to this serious problem.

References

1. Michel M, Gutmann L (1997) Methicillin-resistant Staphylococus aureus and vancomycin-resistant enterococci: therapeutic realities and possibilities. Lancet 349:1901-1906
2. Centers for Disease Control and Prevention (1993) 1989-1993. Nosocomial enterococci resistant to vancomycin. MMWR 42:597-599
3. Hiramatsu K, Hanaki H, Ino T et al (1997) Methicillin-resistant Staphylococcus aureus clinical strain with reduced vancomycin susceptibility. J Antimicrob Chemother 40:135-136
4. Smith TL, Pearson ML, Wilcox KR et al (1999) Emergence of vancomycin resistence in *Staphylococcus aureus*. N Engl J Med 340:493- 501
5. Ackerman BH, Vannier AM, Eudy EB (1992) Analysis of vancomycin time–kill studies with Staphylococcus species by using stripping programs to describe the relationship between concentration and pharmacodynamic response. Antimicrob Agents Chemother 36:1766-1769
6. Di Filippo A, De Gaudio AR, Novelli A et al (1998) Continuous infusion of vancomycin in methicillin-resistant Staphylococcus infection. Chemotherapy 44:63-68
7. Charbonnau P, Harding I,Garaud JJ et al (1994) Teicoplanin: a well-tolerated and easily administered alternative to vancomycin for gram-positive infections in intensive care patients. Intensive Care Med 20:S35-S42
8. Chambers HF (1995) In vitro and in vivo antistaphylococcal activities of L-695,256, a carbapenem with high affinity for the penicillin-binding protein PBP2a. Antimicrob Agents Chemother 39:462-466
9. Ford CW, Hamel JC, Wilson DM et al (1996) In vivo activities of U-100592 and U-100766, novel oxazolidinone antimicrobial agents against experimental bacterial infections. Antimicrob Agents Chemother 40:2820-2823
10. Arthur M, Reynolds P, Courvalin P (1996) Glycopeptide resistance in enterococci. Trends Microbiol 4:401-407
11. Woodford N, Johnson AP, Morrison D, Speller DC (1995) Current perspectives on glycopeptide resistance. Clin Microbiol Rev. 8:585-615

12. Linden PK (1997) Quinupristin/dalfopristin: a new therapeutic alternative for the treatment of vancomycin-resistant *Enterococcus faecium* and other serious Gram-positive infections. Todays Ther Trends 15(2):137-153

13. Nichols RL (1999) Optimal treatment of complicated skin and skin structure infections. J Antimicrob Chemother 44:19-23

14. Fagon J, Patrick H (2000) Treatment of gram-positive nosocomial pneumonia. Prospective randomized comparison of quinupristin/dalfopristin versus vancomycin. Nosocomial Pneumonia Group. Am J Respir Crit Care Med 161:753-762

15. Moellering RC, Linden PK, Reinhardt J et al (1999) The efficacy and safety of quinupristin/dalfopristin for the treatment of infections caused by vancomycin – resistant Enterococcus faecium. J Antimicrob Chemother 44:251-261

16. Rubinstein E, Prokocimer P, Talbot GH (1999) Safety and tolerability of quinupristin/dalfopristin: administration guidelines. J Antimicrob Chemother 44:37-46

Chapter 13

Control of Methicillin-Resistant *Staphylococcus aureus* Outbreaks

S.P. Barrett

Why is there Concern about Methicillin-Resistant *Staphylococcus aureus*

Methicillin-resistant *Staphylococcus aureus* (MRSA) is a term used to describe any strain of *Staphylococcus aureus* that shows resistance to methicillin, thus implying resistance to still-used isoxazolyl penicillins such as flucloxacillin and oxacillin. There are many different strains of MRSA, and one or several may be found in an intensive therapy unit (ITU). Various reasons are put forward for wishing to limit the spread of these organisms. Most convincing is that the spectrum of an empirical antibiotic treatment regime may fail to cover MRSA unless it includes a glycopeptide such as vancomycin or teicoplanin. Another concern is that we are compelled to use what is effectively our last option when we treat MRSA with a glycopeptide. Although it is usually possible to find some alternative drugs active against an MRSA, they tend to be infrequently used agents and there are no general principles of susceptibility to guide empiric therapy. The emergence of glycopeptide-resistant MRSA would undermine the whole of empiric antibiotic treatment and would be of major importance in areas such as the ITU. The recognition in recent years of MRSA with reduced sensitivity to glycopeptides and of enterococci that are frankly resistant shows this concern to be more than just theoretical. A further reason given for needing to control MRSA is that in most cases a patient with an MRSA will have acquired it while in hospital. Clearly, the MRSA will be only one of a wide range of organisms the patient will have acquired during a hospital stay. However, perhaps because they are readily identified and tend to be reported as though they were a single organism, MRSA have acquired a high profile and have entered the public consciousness. Fear of litigation therefore provides another reason for attempting control.

The question of the virulence of MRSA compared with their methicillin-sensitive counterparts (MSSA) has been considered. The vast body of literature now available about MRSA contains almost nothing to suggest that any difference exists. It should be understood that the types of patients who do suffer serious sepsis with MRSA are generally those whose condition is compromised by a range of underlying disorders and various complications of treatment. It is therefore very difficult to make allowance for the highly individual conditions of patients when attempting to compare the outcomes of groups with MRSA and MSSA sepsis. A small number of reports, including some of ITU patients, have suggested that MRSA may be more invasive than MSSA in patients with nasal carriage and that there may be a worse outcome of bacteraemia even with seemingly appropriate antibiotic treatments [1-4]. These exceptional reports should be considered against the background of an absence of such accounts in the wider literature. In addition, as with MSSA, there are likely to be differences in the virulence of individual MRSA strains that may explain such findings. Furthermore, MRSA will obviously have the advantage when best-guess empirical antibiotic therapy does not include a gly-copeptide, and even with 'appropriate' treatment such as vancomycin, it should be noted that this agent is a less potent anti-staphylococcal than those that can be used for MSSA, e.g. flucloxacillin.

MRSA are particularly likely to be of interest in the ITU. Patients who arrive in the ITU are usually the most ill, have various invasive devices, require much direct physical contact and have a history of broad-spectrum antibiotic therapy – all of which will predispose them to colonisation with antibiotic-resistant bacteria. They have frequently been managed in several different clinical specialties during their hospital stay, in any of which MRSA may be prevalent. Furthermore, ITU patients often undergo extensive microbiological investigation and so, if colonised with an MRSA, are more likely than other patients to have it detected [5]. For this reason, ITU which discharge patients to all areas of a hospital are sometimes viewed as a source of the spread of MRSA within a hospital, whereas more correctly it should be recognised that they simply collect the type of patient likely to have acquired an MRSA, and then go to some lengths to detect the organism. At St. Mary's hospital in London, for example, during a 1-year period 14 of 24 ITU patients discovered to have an MRSA were found positive within 48 h of admission to the unit (unpublished observations). Thus, using standard criteria, 58% of ITU patients with an MRSA brought the bacterium into the unit with them. The fact that each admitted case of MRSA was associated with on average less than one detected case of ITU-acquired MRSA could be taken either as a commendation of the care provided by the unit or as evidence that some MRSA at least have little tendency to spread in such circumstances.

Traditional Approach

The means by which attempts to limit MRSA are made will be well known to anyone who has worked on an ITU. In essence, once a patient is found to be MRSA positive, the extent of their carriage is established by screening the usual carrier and other potentially positive sites. As a minimum, this includes the anterior nares, axilla, perineum and any skin breaks such as surgical wounds and intravenous access sites in the ITU patient; catheter urine and respiratory secretions might also be screened. Some centres examine a wide range of other sites, including throat, hairline, wrists and interdigital clefts. Care is taken to dispose promptly of dressings, secretions, bed linen etc. and equipment used on the patient will, where possible, be 'decontaminated' before being used on others. To prevent staff becoming MRSA carriers or else acting as passive vectors for transmission of MRSA, they should use protective clothing, which is usually limited to disposable gloves and aprons, and antiseptic handwash agents will be used. In an ordinary ward context, patients with an MRSA will be transferred to an isolation room for nursing, but the constraints of ITU often make this impossible. If the carrier sites prove positive, the patient will be treated with an antiseptic 'protocol' over a period of days. Ideally, patients treated with such antiseptic protocols will be checked a few days after finishing to determine whether their MRSA has been cleared. A considerable number of variations of decontamination protocols exist, but usually antiseptic wash solutions (e.g. chlorhexidine, iodine, hexachlorophene) are applied to areas of skin carriage, and MRSA in other superficial sites such as the anterior nares or conjunctiva will be treated with antiseptic ointments. Mupirocin is favoured for nasal carriage providing the MRSA is sensitive to it, and topical antibiotics such as neomycin and bacitracin can be applied to certain other sites. An infection, as opposed to colonisation, with an MRSA will naturally warrant appropriate antibiotic treatment.

The above represents the textbook response to finding a single patient with an MRSA. If it appears that the MRSA has been acquired by at least one other patient in the unit or area, the traditional response is to initiate outbreak investigation and control. In its most extreme form, this involves closing the ward and screening all patients and staff for MRSA carriage. Any patient found to be MRSA positive will be treated in the same fashion as the index case, perhaps being 'cohort' nursed in the same multiple-bed room as others found to be positive, but preferably with all such patients being removed to a dedicated isolation unit. If it is impossible to avoid nursing MRSA-positive and MRSA-negative patients in the same unit, they must be physically segregated and separate nursing teams should be designated – one dealing with the MRSA positive patients, and one with those who are MRSA negative. Any staff member found to be carrying an MRSA will be sent off work with antiseptic treatments. They will be allowed to return to work only when follow-up screening swabs, taken on one or more occasions depending on local policy, show that the MRSA has gone. When all patients and staff have been cleared of MRSA, the unit will be subjected to thorough cleaning in an attempt to remove MRSA that may have contaminated the environment. Thereafter it will reopen.

Practical Problems

The above approach to controlling MRSA was first described in a European context in guidelines produced by a U.K. working party of the Hospital Infection Society and British Society for Antimicrobial Chemotherapy in 1986 [6]. It will be immediately apparent that such a vigorous approach to MRSA will very rarely be practicable and in an ITU, given the intensity of activity and the high dependency of patients, will be all but impossible. The closure of an ITU clearly has major consequences for the acute activity of a hospital and will only be undertaken in the most compelling of circumstances.

The working party which drew up the above guidelines recognised the difficulties of an ideal approach and gave details for the more practical management of MRSA patients, such as the use of dedicated staff for patients undergoing cohort nursing and how to deal with trolleys, ambulances etc. While dealing with MRSA in this manner might be contemplated in areas where these organisms are encountered extremely rarely, it is clearly out of the question to do so when they are found more often. For example, the 1992 European Prevalence of Infection in Intensive Care (EPIC) study [7] showed that at least 8% of patients in European ITU could be expected to have MRSA. If the extremes of MRSA management recommendations were applied in this situation, many ITU would effectively cease to function. Successive revisions of the British working party MRSA control guidelines [6, 8] have had to acknowledge the relentless increase of prevalence of these organisms, and the approach adopted by the most recent version has been modified to accept that MRSA are now endemic in many areas. Rather than seeking to eliminate MRSA overall, the guidelines now suggest that attention is focused on areas accommodating vulnerable patients – such as ITU – which it is suggested should continue a vigorous approach to MRSA, while recognising the same will not occur in other parts of the hospital. However, progressive recognition of the realities of MRSA prevalence by guideline writers does not make matters more manageable for ITU. To comply with current recommendations, given the frequency with which ITU receive MRSA patients – who may be admitted as unrecognised carriers – would require extra resources in terms of personnel and environment, which clearly are not forthcoming.

Results of the Traditional Approach

History provides many examples of infectious agents that have come and gone apparently unrelated to deliberate human endeavours, e.g. encephalitis lethargica and European tuberculosis before the advent of bacille Calmette-Guérin (BCG). Thus, activities undertaken with the aim of controlling an infectious agent may be responsible for its subsequent reduction, or else this may have been simply a coincidence. In the Middle Ages, people may have believed the rituals they practised to rid themselves of repeated epidemics of bubonic plague were at times successful, but we would probably not concur today. Reports of success in controlling MRSA should be recognised as exceptional given the progressive increase in numbers overall, and the possibility of publication bias should also be borne in mind. However, a few authors have described apparent success that was later found to be short-lived. For example, Cox et al. [9, 10] reported how an outbreak of MRSA was brought under control at considerable expense and disruption and how control was eventually lost. Similarly, Farrington et al. [11] described the pressures that appeared to cause an eventual loss of control of MRSA. A similar thing appears to have happened in Western Australia [12, 13] and the results of other studies have caused authors overtly to question the value of MRSA control measures [14, 15].

Although some still advocate approaching MRSA control by methods such as those given in the current British guidelines, it is clear that what has been done so far has failed. The most convincing manifestation of failure is the ever-increasing numbers of isolates of MRSA reported by most countries each year. Although it can certainly be said that the detailed measures advocated by control programmes (e.g. isolation nursing, screening for carriers) seem reasonable things to do if

MRSA control is to be attempted, it does need to be recognised that there is very little by way of scientific evidence to prove their worth. In fairness, it should also be said that it would be impossibly difficult to design studies to prove or disprove their value. However, consideration of whether or not these control measures are intrinsically sound may not be relevant. For example, Clark et al. [16] found that only 46% of 261 patients who should have been screened for MRSA had any screening samples taken, and less than half of these were screened correctly. At St. Mary's Hospital in London, an attempt to examine for MRSA in all the patients entering the ITU during a 1-year period resulted in 59% being screened, and in a vascular surgical ward of the hospital, where the ward staff themselves had suggested screening all patients admitted, only 23% were in fact examined (unpublished observations). A study in Wales showed that, although some hospitals had stringent written policies for the control of MRSA, staff admitted they were unable to comply with them [15]. Thus, whatever may be the intrinsic merits of suggested control measures, they are clearly valueless if staff do not apply them in practice.

It would be unfortunate enough if attempts at controlling MRSA represented only futile expenditure of effort. However, there are also substantial costs in applying recommended control measures [17]. These are not only financial [9], but may also interfere with patient care and involve human factors such as isolation and cause suffering for elderly patients in particular [18]. Staff may feel stigmatised and demoralised; at St. Mary's Hospital some years ago, the reopening of a surgical ward following an MRSA outbreak was delayed because a substantial number of nurses had resigned during the closure. Given the clear disadvantages to outbreak control programmes, and the statistics that give no reason to believe they have done anything to check the advance of MRSA, it is difficult to make a convincing argument for continuing with them.

It should be noted that mention is sometimes made of certain areas where MRSA control policies are held to have been successful. Most commonly mentioned in this context are Western Australia, the Netherlands and Denmark. Clearly each country, and even each hospital, will have unique features that may have a bearing on its experience with MRSA. Western Australia is sparsely populated, and it was considered that a strictly applied screening programme for all hospital admissions from outside the state had prevented the introduction of MRSA [11]. This may indeed be correct, but later reports have noted an inexorable increase in numbers of cases of a local strain of MRSA in Western Australia. The Netherlands appears never to have significant numbers of MRSA and enforces a screening policy for hospital transfers from abroad. The Netherlands is able to quote some of the few success stories where hospital outbreaks of an MRSA appear to have been overcome [19]. Denmark provides a curious history of MRSA being widespread some years before they were prevalent in most other countries. Subsequently, these MRSA all but disappeared, but Danish workers of the time did not claim this as a success for infection control measures; rather they suggested changes in antibiotic prescribing practices might have been responsible [20].

How does Methicillin-Resistant *Staphylococcus aureus* Spread?

These national differences in experience with MRSA control may in fact be of importance in understanding how to deal with MRSA. Firstly, it appears that the essentials of MRSA control programmes – isolation and treatment of affected individuals, screening and treating carriers, outbreak management – are the same in all countries. Yet some countries practice these measures with apparent success, while others practise them and fail. These seemingly vastly different results of the same control activities must cast serious doubt on their true role in influencing levels of MRSA and raise the possibility that other unrecognised factors are more important. Furthermore, although still relatively rarely, MRSA are increasingly to be found in the non-hospital population, and ever increasing international travel means that unrecognised cases must pass between countries and inevitably on occasion be admitted to hospital. Yet in the hospitals of some countries MRSA has become endemic, while in others it is scarcely to be found. Hoefnagels-Schuermans et al. [21] found 5% of patients had MRSA on admission to their hospital, but the repeated introduction of these community strains did not result in spread. In contrast, their ITU, which had an MRSA problem, was affected by a small number of strains that appeared particularly transmissible. This contrasts with the experience quoted above of the St. Mary's ITU in London, where spread of MRSA appeared minimal. Strain differences in propensity to spread may therefore be one of the factors determining MRSA levels. Other factors that may contribute have not been formally studied, e.g. understaffing has been correlated with increased transmission [22, 23] of MRSA and other staphylococci in neonatal intensive care units, and it would be of interest to compare staff to patient ratios in ITU in different countries. Health service expenditure, antibiotic policies and hospital design are other factors that may all play as yet unrecognised roles in determining experience with MRSA in different countries.

The mathematical model of Cooper et al. [24] has suggested that difference in strain transmissibility is a major determinant of the spread of MRSA in hospital units. Other factors were also shown by this analysis to have an important bearing on levels of MRSA. Short stay (i.e. high patient throughput) gave greater opportunities for repeated introduction and the establishment of MRSA. Handwashing was also shown to be important, with even a small increase in the frequency of handwashing leading to an important reduction in the spread of MRSA.

Of course, the exact mechanism of transmission of an MRSA from one patient to another is almost never known. Cooper's model [24], like others, has made the assumption that the usual route of transmission is by staff acting as a passive vector for transfer. Patients themselves are considered unlikely to spread MRSA to each other by direct physical contact, and airborne and fomite spread are discounted. Whether the latter are reasonable assumptions can be debated, but the model does at least suggest the potential importance of factors that have so far received less attention than they might.

The role of carriers in spreading MRSA is, to judge by the importance placed by control guidelines on seeking them out, traditionally considered important. This assumption, too, has come to be questioned in recent years. It must firstly be understood that the finding of an MRSA on either a staff member or a patient is quite likely to represent transient or temporary carriage. Staff carriers have on occasion contributed to the spread of MRSA, but an MRSA recovered from a staff member is generally unrelated to patient strains both within the ITU setting and without [25, 26, 27]. Staff and patients found to be MRSA positive on screening are of course always given some form of treatment and not merely followed until their MRSA disappears spontaneously. The natural history of leaving untreated those who screen positive for MRSA will therefore not be familiar to most infection control workers. However, there is at least one report to suggest that MRSA clearance is little influenced by the 'decontamination' regimes that are used [15].

Conversely, other factors that may be of importance in the spread of MRSA are relatively neglected in current control practices. Work done more than 40 years ago suggested that certain carriers of *Staphylococcus aureus* were much more likely to disseminate organisms into their environment than others [28], and similar, more recent work [26, 29] has indicated that respiratory carriers with upper respiratory tract infection are particularly likely to spread MRSA. Measuring such events is, of course, much more complicated than the screening swabs that are usually recommended and is therefore not done, even though the identification of individuals who are shedding MRSA excessively might aid the control of some outbreaks.

Are Alternative Approaches Worth Considering?

There can be little argument that the methods tried so far have at best delayed the progress of MRSA. Rather than continue with them and cause difficulties for our patients and ourselves, it is time to consider alternative approaches. The spread of MRSA tells us that organisms are passing between patients in hospitals. It is unlikely this can ever be prevented, but we can at least try to reduce the opportunities for transmission and the consequences of its occurring. Reduction in transmission, as suggested by the model of Cooper et al. [24], could yield important benefits at the simple cost of increased handwashing. This seemingly obvious activity may not be taking place when poor design of units prevents ready access to wash basins and when clinicians are prepared to be quoted as viewing handwashing as unnecessary [30]. The need for the current U.K. initiative [31] to improve handwashing is a sad reflection of the state which matters have reached. While patients' acquisition of micro-organisms is ultimately inevitable, we should seek to ensure that those acquired in hospital are as harmless as possible. Antibiotic resistance, such as displayed by MRSA, complicates patients' treatment, and antibiotic resistance should therefore be avoided. It is generally believed that control of antibiotic usage is the only means currently available for achieving this. A few studies do support this. Most MRSA are now resistant to ciprofloxacin, and a recent study by Manhold and colleagues [32] suggested ITU patients treated with ciprofloxacin were prone to superinfection with *S. aureus*, including MRSA. This led the authors to recommend that ciprofloxacin should be used in combination with an agent with better activity against gram-positive bacteria. The classic work by Price and Sleigh [33] in a

Scottish ITU showed that antibiotic resistance could be reduced by restricting usage of certain agents. More recent studies have supported these observations in both ITU [34] and other acute intensive units [35].

Conclusions

MRSA are rightly considered as hospital-acquired organisms that may be responsible for excess morbidity in the compromised patient. However, we should recognise that they represent just one type of hospital-acquired bacterium, which can act as a marker for cross-infection in hospital. The excessive interest that has focused on these organisms and which has failed to contain them has been a disservice to the wider aims of hospital infection control. Rather than continue to fail with policies of attempted containment, future efforts should consider MRSA within the overall context of hospital-acquired infection and should investigate alternative approaches such as the identification of factors which allow MRSA to flourish.

References

1. Romero-Vivas J, Rubio M, Fernandez C, Picazo JJ (1995) Mortality associated with nosocomial bacteremia due to methicillin-resistant Staphylococcus aureus. Clin Infect Dis 21:1417-1423
2. Catchpole C, Wise R, Fraise A (1997) MRSA bacteraemia. J Hosp Infect 35:159-161
3. Pujol M, Peña C, Pallares R et al (1996) Nosocomial Staphylococcus aureus bacteremia among nasal carriers of methicillin-resistant and methicillin-susceptible strains. Am J Med 100:509-516
4. Barrett SP (1997) MRSA pathogenicity and bacteraemia. J Hosp Infect 37:171-172
5. Barrett SP, Mellor JA (1990) Living with EMRSA-1. J Hosp Infect 15:103-104
6. Working Party of the Hospital Infection Society and British Society for Antimicrobial Chemotherapy (1986) Guidelines for the control of epidemic methicillin-resistant Staphylococcus aureus. J Hosp Infect 7:193-201
7. Vincent JL, Bihari DJ, Suter PM et al (1995) The prevalence of nosocomial infection in intensive care units in Europe. Results of the European Prevalence of Infection in Intensive Care (EPIC) study. JAMA 274:639-644
8. Working Party of the BSAC, HIS and ICNA (1998) Revised guidelines for the control of methicillin-resistant Staphylococcus aureus. J Hosp Infect 39:253-290
9. Cox RA, Conquest C, Mallaghan C, Marples RR (1995) A major outbreak of methicillin-resistant Staphylococcus aureus caused by a new phage-type (EMRSA-16). J Hosp Infect 29:87-106
10. Cox RA, Conquest C (1997) Strategies for the management of healthcare staff colonized with epidemic methicillin-resistant Staphylococcus aureus. J Hosp Infect 35:117-127
11. Farrington M, Redpath C, Trundle C et al (1998) Winning the battle but losing the war: methicillin-resistant Staphylococcus aureus (MRSA) infection at a teaching hospital. Q J Med 91:539-548
12. Riley TV, Rouse IL (1995) Methicillin-resistant Staphylococcus aureus in Western Australia 1983-1992. J Hosp Infect 29:177-188
13. Torvaldsen S, Roberts C, Riley TV (1999) The continuing evolution of methicillin-resis-

tant Staphylococcus aureus in Western Australia. Infect Control Hosp Epidemiol 20:133-135

14. Barrett SP, Teare EL, Sage R (1993) Methicillin-resistant Staphylococcus aureus in three adjacent Health Districts of south-east England 1986-91. J Hosp Infect 24:313-325

15. Morgan M, Evans-Williams D, Salmon R et al (2000) The population impact of MRSA in a country: the national survey of MRSA in Wales. J Hosp Infect 44:227-239

16. Clark B, Fryer J, Emslie A et al (1999) Why is something as important as screening for MRSA so difficult to achieve? P589 presented the 21st International Congress of Chemotherapy, July 4-7, Birmingham

17. Barrett SP, Mummery RV, Chattopadhyay B (1998) Trying to control MRSA causes more problems than it solves. J Hosp Infect 39:85-93

18. Taylor ME, Oppenheim BA (1998) Hospital-acquired infection in elderly patients. J Hosp Infect 38:245-260

19. Vanderbroucke-Grauls CM (1993) Control of methicillin-resistant Staphyloocccus aureus in the Netherlands. In: Coello R, Casewell MW (eds) Methicillin-resistant Staphylococcus aureus. Wells, Kent, pp 87-106

20. Rosdahl VT, Knudsen AM (1991) The decline of methicillin resistance among Danish Staphylococcus aureus strains. Infect Control Hosp Epidemiol 12:83-88

21. Hoefnagels-Schuermans A, Borremans A, Peetermans W et al (1997) Origin and transmission of methicillin-resistant Staphylococcus aureus in an endemic situation: differences between geriatric and intensive-care patients. J Hosp Infect 36:209-222

22. Haley RW, Bregman DA (1982) The role of understaffing and overcrowding in recurrent outbreaks of staphylococcal infection in a neonatal special-care unit. J Infect Dis 145:875-885

23. Haley RW, Cushion NB, Tenover FC et al (1995) Eradication of endemic methicillin-resistant Staphylococcus aureus infections from a neonatal intensive care unit. J Infect Dis 171:614-624

24. Cooper BS, Medley GF, Scott GM (1999) Preliminary analysis of the transmission dynamics of nosocomial infections: stochastic and management effects. J Hosp Infect 43:131-147

25. Lessing MPA, Jordens JZ, Bowler ICJ (1997) When should healthcare workers be screened for methicillin-resistant Staphylococcus aureus? J Hosp Infect 34:205-210

26. Boyce JM, Opal SM, Potter-Bynoe G, Medeiros AA (1993) Spread of methicillin-resistant Staphylococcus aureus in a hospital after exposure to a health care worker with chronic sinusitis. Clin Infect Dis 17:496-504

27. Mueller-Premru M, Muzlovic I (1998) Typing of consecutive methicillin-resistant Staphylococcus aureus isolates from intensive care unit patients and staff with pulsed-field gel electrophoresis. Int J Antimicrob Agents 10:309-312

28. Hare R, Thomas CGA (1956) The transmission of Staphylococcus aureus. Br Med J ii:840-846

29. Sheretz RJ, Reagan DR, Hampton KD et al (1996) A cloud adult: the Staphylococcus aureus-virus interaction revisited. Ann Intern Med 124:539-547

30. Weeks A. (1999) Why I don't wash my hands between each patient contact. Br Med J 319:518

31. Teare EL, Cookson B, French GL et al (1999) UK handwashing initiative. J Hosp Infect 43:1-3

32. Manhold C, von Rolbicki U, Brase R et al (1998) Outbreaks of Staphylococcus aureus infections during treatment of late onset pneumonia with ciprofloxacin in a prospective, randomized study. Intens Care Med 24:1327-1230

33. Price DJE, Sleigh JD (1970) Control of infection due to Klebsiella aerogenes in a neurosurgical unit by withdrawal of all antibiotics. Lancet ii:1213-1215

34. Mohammedi I, Duperret S, Védrinne JM et al (1998) Du bon usage des antibiotiques en réanimation: résultats d'un programme de rationalisation de la prescription. Ann Fr Anaesthiol Réan 17:27-31

35. Reed CS, Barrett SP, Threlfall J, Cheasty T (1995) Control of infection with multiple resistant bacteria in a hospital renal unit: the value of plasmid characterization. Epidemiol Infect 115:61-70

Chapter 14

Oral Vancomycin in the Control of MRSA Outbreaks in the ICU

M.A. DE LA CAL, E. CERDÁ, M. CALDERÓN, P. GARCÍA-HIERRO, H.K.F. VAN SAENE

Introduction

Methicillin-resistant *Staphylococcus aureus* (MRSA) is a serious problem, both clinically and epidemiologically. Systemic vancomycin is the cornerstone for the therapy of invasive infections due to MRSA. However, vancomycin is potentially toxic and there is an increasing fear that microorganisms resistant to vancomycin such as vancomycin-resistant enterococci (VRE) [1] and vancomycin intermediate *Staphylococcus aureus* (VISA) will emerge [2].

The traditional approach to the control of MRSA includes surveillance of the nasal carriage, topical mupirocin to eradicate nasal carriage, handwashing and isolation to prevent MRSA transmission [3-5], and systemic vancomycin in case of suspected infection. Despite occasional reports of local success, the steadily increasing prevalence of strains of MRSA shows that attempts to limit their spread do not work [6].

Outbreaks due to multi-resistant *Klebsiella* sp have been brought under control using oral polymyxin/tobramycin [7,8] mainly because this approach prevents the carriage and overgrowth of multi-resistant gram-negative bacilli in the digestive tract, which is the main reservoir of flora resistant to antimicrobials. On the other hand, oral vancomycin has been reported to effectively clear *Clostridium difficile* [9] and methicillin-sensitive *Staphylococcus aureus* from the gut without any harmful side effects. In line with this experience we designed a new protocol based on the use of topical vancomycin in the throat and gut, with the aim of abolishing the digestive tract carrier state of MRSA so as to control an MRSA outbreak.

A prospective 39-month study was undertaken to evaluate the efficacy and safety of topical vancomycin both as treatment of the carrier state once carriage was detected and as prophylaxis of the carrier state, in the control of endemic MRSA.

Patients and Methods

Patients

Patients expected to require mechanical ventilation for at least 3 days were enrolled in this study over a period of 3 years and 3 months (1 July, 1996 to 30 September, 1999). The setting of the study was a medical/surgical intensive care unit (ICU) in the Hospital Universitario de Getafe. All patients were consecutively enrolled.

Design and Interventions

This prospective study comprises three different periods. Period I was observational, from 1 July, 1996 to 20 April, 1997. A continuous surveillance of clinical samples positive to MRSA was implemented. The clinical samples were taken on clinical indication. Patients with positive clinical samples were isolated in a single-bedded room. Systemic vancomycin was administered only in case of suspected infection.

The next two periods were interventional. In addition to diagnostic samples, surveillance samples of nose, throat, rectum, tracheostomy, and pressure sores were obtained on admission, and afterwards once weekly. In period II from 1 May, 1997 to 30 September, 1998 oral vancomycin was started once carriage was detected. In period III from 1 October, 1998 to 30 September 1999, oral vancomycin was added to the selective digestive decontamination protocol as prophylaxis of the MRSA carrier state when patients were intubated.

A 4 % paste was applied topically into the oropharyngeal cavity, onto the tracheostoma and the pressure sores four times a day. A vancomycin suspension, 500 mg, was administered via the nasogastric tube four times a day.

The skin was washed with 4% chlorhexidine twice a week. All patients who were found to be carriers of multi-resistant microorganisms were isolated in separate rooms.

Endpoints

Primary endpoints: cumulative incidence of patients in whom clinical samples were positive for MRSA 48 h after admission in the ICU.

Secondary endpoints were (1) cumulative incidence of patients who were negative for MRSA in the surveillance samples on admission, and acquired MRSA later in the ICU; and (2) the percentage of samples which were positive for VRE both clinically and during surveillance in period II and period III.

Definitions

A new case was defined as a patient who was not known as an MRSA carrier and who had an MRSA-positive sample, surveillance sample and/or clinical sample.

Surveillance samples included swabs obtained from the oropharynx and rectum, to detect digestive tract carriage. A surveillance set also included a nasal swab, and in patients with tracheostoma and/or pressure sores, samples from the stoma and sores. Surveillance samples were taken immediately on admission and once weekly thereafter. A patient was considered to have imported MRSA when the first set of surveillance swabs were positive for MRSA on admission. In all other cases MRSA was considered to be ICU acquired.

Clinical samples included those from tracheal aspirate, blood, urine, wounds, and invasive lines that were not taken routinely on arrival but only on clinical indication. A patient with a clinical sample yielding MRSA within 48 h was considered to have imported bacteria. Clinical samples positive for MRSA after 2 days were due to acquisition in the ICU.

Overgrowth was defined as the presence of $\geq 10^7$ cfu/ml of MRSA per milliliter of surveillance samples . As the presence of MRSA in clinical sample is abnormal, the term *positive clinical sample* was used in this study rather than infection or colonization in order to avoid the inherent bias related to the diagnosis of some infections such as pneumonia.

Statistical analysis

Continuous variables were compared using the Student-t-test or Wilconson's test when appropriate. Discrete variables were compared using Chi-square or Fisher's exact test.

Results

Patients

The general characteristics of the patients were similar in the three periods. About a quarter of all admissions were expected to require mechanical ventilation for more than 3 days. The age was 61 ($\pm$ 18) years, the average SAPS II was 39 ($\pm$ 13), the length of stay was 19 ($\pm$ 18), and the mortality was 29 %. About half of the population had an underlying medical condition, one third of the patients required intensive care following surgery, and 15% were trauma cases.

Acquired Positive Clinical Samples

Topical vancomycin treatment either as therapy of carriage or as prophylaxis of carriage of MRSA significantly reduced the cumulative incidence of acquired positive clinical samples in 14% and 2%, respectively, in comparison with the historical control group of 31% (Table. 1).

A total of 44 patients (31 %) had 63 acquired clinical positive samples for MRSA during period I; 37 patients (14 %) had 55 during period II, whereas five patients (2 %) had a total of 5 during period III (Table 1).

Finally, the number of positive clinical samples per patient was significantly lower in the prophylaxis group than in the first and the second groups (Fig. 1). The two main types of positive clinical samples obtained during the study were from tracheal aspirates and intravascular catheters.

Impact of Topical Vancomycin on MRSA Carriage Developed in the ICU

A total of 65 (25%) patients were found to be MRSA carriers during the application of topical vancomycin to treat the carrier state (period II), whereas 58 (28%)

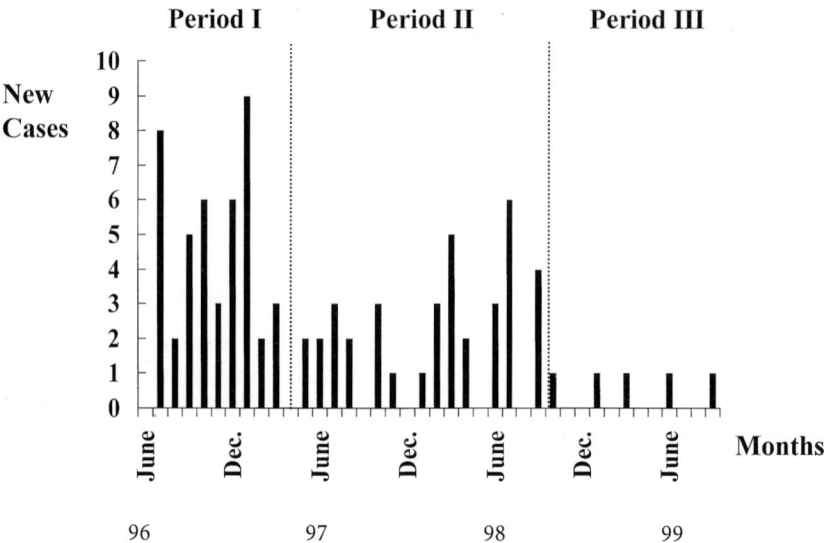

Fig. 1. Acquired MRSA-positive clinical samples

Table 1. Newly acquired cases

Cases	Period I [a]	Period II	Period III
Patients (*n*)	140	258	206
Patients with positive surveillance and/or clinical samples (*n*)	44	58 (22%)	25 (12%)
Patients with positive clinical samples (*n*)	44 (31%)	37 (14%)*	5 (2%)*
Patients with positive surveillance samples with overgrowth ($\geq 10^7$ cfu/ml) (%)	—	52%	0%*
Patients with positive surveillance samples < 10^5 cfu/ml (%)	—	6%	55%
Positive clinical samples (*n*)	63	55	5
Tracheal aspirate	30	26	1
Intravascular catheters	16	18	3
Blood cultures	11	5	0
Surgical wounds	2	3	1
Urine	3	1	0
Intraventricular catheter	1	1	0

[a] In period I only clinical samples were reported
* *p*< 0.001

patients carried MRSA during vancomycin administration to prevent the carrier state (period III). Fourteen patients had MRSA upon admission, and 51 acquired MRSA in the ICU during period II. During period III, 35 patients imported MRSA and 23 acquired the strain while in the ICU. Significantly fewer patients acquired MRSA when topical vancomycin was immediately given to patients on arrival to the ICU. Out of 258 patients, 75% had overgrowth in period II. In contrast, in period III comprising 206 patients, only 12 patients showed overgrowth ($p<0.01$).

Safety of Topical Vancomycin: Emergence of VRE

There was a VRE outbreak affecting 13 patients form April 1998 to August 1999. A total of five patients showed clinical samples positive to VRE, two on arrival and three who developed positive samples during their stay in the ICU. The outbreak spontaneously disappeared without any change in policy.

All MRSA isolated from clinical samples showed a minimal inhibitory concentration under 4 mg per milliliter.

Discussion

The answers to the endpoints of the study are: (1) oral vancomycin both as treatment and prevention of throat and gut carriage leads to significantly fewer clinical samples yielding MRSA; (2) oral vancomycin successfully controlled throat and gut overgrowth, although prophylaxis was more effective; and (3) oral vancomycin was safe in terms of selecting VRE.

Form the point of view of the study design, the substantial sample size of the study as well as the long-term follow-up are the major strengths of the prospective trial. The non-randomized design does not allow firm conclusions about the causal relationship between intervention and outcomes to be made. However, in the control of outbreaks, a sequential design is a well-accepted methodology. Different populations and changes in the level of hygiene are often mentioned as the main drawbacks of sequential comparisons. In this study, there were more patients who carried MRSA on admission during period III than in period II. The level of hygiene apparently did not alter as the number of clinical sample positive for MRSA of exogenous development were similar during the two study periods.

The efficacy of topical vancomycin in throat and gut in this study can be explained by the following findings. Gastrointestinal carriage of MRSA may represent a larger source [10-12] for spreading than the nasal cavity. Studies report MRSA concentrations of 10^8 cfu/g of feces, compared with 10^2 cfu per cm^2 of nasal mucosal surface. That concept may partly explain the failures and the high rates of relapses of topical mupirocin in the control of MRSA.

Topical vancomycin administered to the population at risk immediately on admission was more effective in the reduction of clinical samples positive for MRSA because that mode of application prevented carriage and subsequent overgrowth of MRSA. In contrast, topical vancomycin for the eradication of established carriage implies an inherent delay, allowing overgrowth and cross-transmission.

Reinforcement of traditional measures, including isolation, hand washing and gloving was sufficient in the control of the VRE outbreak. We do not believe there is a link between the topical vancomycin protocol and the emergence of the VRE outbreak for two reasons: the outbreak was stopped after 5 months despite continuous oral vancomycin treatment for more than 2 years. Most VRE outbreaks are described in ICUs that have never used topical vancomycin and often those outbreaks last for long periods. Systemic third-generation cephalosporin, ciprofloxacin, antibiotics with potent antianaerobic activity, and vancomycin [1, 13, 14] have been reported to promote enterococcal overgrowth, following disruption of the normal gut flora. The recommended empirical treatments for lower airway infections [15, 16] often include combinations of systemic antibiotics covering both gram-negative and gram-positive microorganisms that promote VRE outbreaks. In our study, the fact that one VRE outbreak was controlled in a short time and without relapse 2 years later may be due to the high fecal levels of up to 3000 mg/g of feces following the oral administration of 2 g of vancomycin that prevent VRE strains overgrowth [17, 18].

Results of this study should be carefully considered by those epidemiologists and intensive care specialists coping with the control of MRSA outbreaks in the ICU.

References

1. HICPAP (1994) Recommendations for preventing the spread of vancomycin resistance. Recommendations of the Hospital Infection Control Practices Advisory Committee (HICPAP). MMWR 44:1-12
2. Smith TL, Pearson ML, Wilcox KR et al (1999) Emergence of vancomycin resistance in Staphylococcus aureus. N Engl J Med 340:493-501
3. Boyce JM, Jackson MM, Pugliese G et al (1994) Methicillin-resistant *Staphylococcus aureus* (MRSA): a briefing for acute care hospitals and nursing facilities. The AHA technical panel on infections within Hospitals. Infect Control Hosp Epidemiol 15:105-115
4. Wenzel R, Reagan DR, Bertino JS et al (1998) Methicillin-resistant *Staphylococcus aureus* outbreak: a consensus panel's definition and management guidelines. AJIC 26:102-110
5. Working Party Report (1998) Revised guidelines for the control of methicillin-resistant infection in hospitals. J Hosp Infect 39:253-290
6. Barrett SP, Mummery RV (1998) Trying to control MRSA causes more problems than it solves. J Hosp Infect 39:85-93
7. Brun-Buisson C, Legrand P, Rauss A et al (1989) Intestinal decontamination for control of nosocomial multiresistant Gram-negative bacilli. Ann Intern Med 110:873-881
8. Taylor ME, Oppenheim BA (1991) Selective decontamination of the gastrointestinal tract as an infection control measure. J Hosp Infect 17:271-278
9. Fekety R (1997) Guidelines for the diagnosis and management of *Chlostridium difficile* associated diarrhea and colitis. American College of Gastroenterology, Practice Parameters Committee. Am J Gastroenterol 92:739-750
10. Crossley K, Landesman B, Zaske D (1979) An outbreak of infections caused by strains of Staphylococcus aureus resistant to methicillin and aminoglycosides. II. Epidemiologic studies. J Infect Dis 139: 280-287
11. Rimland D, Roberson B (1986) Gastrointestinal carriage of methicillin-resistant Staphylococcus aureus. J Clin Microbiol 24:137-138

12. Brady LM, Thomson M, Palmer MA, Harkness JL (1990) Successful control of endemic MRSA in a cardiothoracic surgical unit. Med J Aust 152:240-252
13. Bonten MJM, Hyaden MK, Nathan C et al (1996) Epidemiology of colonisation of patients and environment with vancomycin-resistant enterococci. Lancet 348:1615-1619
14. Linden PK, Miller CB (1999) Vancomycin-resistant enterococci: the clinical effect of a common nosocomial pathogen. Diagn Microbiol Infect Dis 33:113-120
15. ATS guidelines (1995) Hospital-acquired pneumonia in adults: diagnosis, assessment, initial therapy, and prevention: a consensus statement. Am J Respir Crit Care Med 153:1711-1725
16. Barlett JG, Breiman RF, Mandell LA, File TM Jr (1998) Community-acquired pneumonia: guidelines for management. Clin Infect Dis 26:811-838
17. Tedesco F, Markham R, Gurwith M, et al (1978) Oral vaycomycin for antibiotic associated pseudomembranous colitis. Lancet ii:226-228
18. Khan MY, Hall WH (1966) Staphylococcal enterocolitis – treatment with oral vancomycin. Ann Intern Med 65:1-8

Chapter 15

Control of *Acinetobacter* Outbreaks with Oral Polymyxin

M. Sánchez, M. Álvarez

Introduction

Acinetobacter (*A.*) *baumannii* has emerged in recent years as an important noso-comial pathogen, both because it frequently causes severe infections [1, 2] with multidrug-resistant strains [3-8], and because it is involved in multiple epidemic outbreaks in intensive care units (ICU) [9-13] and general hospital wards [4, 10, 14, 15]. In spite of intense efforts to control and prevent colonization and infection, *A. baumannii* has become endemic in ICU in Spain [10, 16-18] and many other countries [2-4, 8, 9, 15, 19-21].

The clinical relevance of preventing and controlling *A. baumannii* colonization and infection has been illustrated by Fagon [22] in a matched-control study performed in 48 patients with ventilator-associated pneumonia (VAP). Compared to the control group, patients suffering from VAP with *Acinetobacter* or *Pseudomonas* spp. had a risk ratio of dying of 2.5. Lortholary et al. [21] later confirmed that the acquisition of *A. baumannii* during ICU stay, together with a high APACHE II score, is independently associated with mortality and significantly prolongs ICU stay. In a study by Garrouste-Orgeas et al. [23], who compared colonized with infected with noncolonized patients, carriage and infection with multi-resistant *A. baumannii* and/or *Klebsiella pneumoniae* were associated with increased mortality in patients with a SAPS score lower than 16. Similar data have recently been reported in a matched-control study from Spain performed by García Garmendia in Seville [16]. In that study, 75 patients who acquired *A. baumannii* during their ICU stay had a crude ICU mortality of 49%, compared to 19% in the control group. In study patients, mortality increased from 33% to 58% in the subset developing infection, and reached 70% in patients with respiratory infections. Compared to the control group, the diagnosis of respiratory infection with *A. baumannii* was associated with a risk rate of death of 4.0.

Distribution and Colonization Pattern of Acinetobacter

Acinetobacter is ubiquitous in nature and may colonize the skin of healthy individuals [24, 25]. However, the natural reservoir for those species causing nosocomial infections has not been identified [25]. In hospitalized patients *Acinetobacter* spp. have been identified on almost any epithelium [11, 12, 17, 21,

23, 26], depending on the design of the sampling protocol. It colonizes ICU patients during outbreaks and in nonoutbreak situations and can be recovered from the upper and lower respiratory tract, the digestive tract, from the oropharynx to the rectum, as well as from different areas of the skin, such as the nose, axilla, and groin.

Pathophysiology of Acinetobacter Infections

It is generally accepted that most ICU-acquired infections are of secondary endogenous development [27]. Garrouste-Orgeas et al. [23], for example, observed that 91% of ICU-acquired nosocomial infections were preceded by oropharyngeal and/or rectal carriage. According to this classification [27], a potentially pathogenic microorganism (PPM) is acquired by cross-colonization via the hands of health care personnel and colonizes the aerodigestive tract of a critically ill patient. The PPM may also arise from the endogenous flora of the patient as a result of selective antibiotic pressure. This pathophysiologic sequence of events has repeatedly been demonstrated for gram-positive [28, 29] and gram-negative bacteria [30, 31], as well as for fungal infections [32]. Typically, the pathogenic microorganism can be demonstrated in surveillance cultures obtained several days after ICU admission [23]. It may spread to the upper and lower airway and colonize the digestive tract, as well as surgical and burn wounds, decubitus ulcers, and tracheostomas [8]. A subset of colonized patients develop infection which is preceded by several days to weeks of colonization [12, 17, 23, 23, 26]. The risk factors for infection in colonized patients are poorly understood, but may be associated with the number of sites that are colonized [32] and the density of the inoculum.

In contrast, secondary exogenous infections are infrequent [23], or even anecdotal, in the ICU setting. Examples are infections due to direct inoculation of microorganisms, without prior aerodigestive colonization, such as an episode of nosocomial pneumonia after bronchoscopy with a contaminated bronchoscope.

Colonization is the most important risk factor for ICU-acquired infection with the colonizing microorganism [30, 32]. This concept also holds true for *Acinetobacter* spp. Timsit et al. [11], for example, reported that 11 (27%) of 41 colonized patients developed infection with *A. baumannii*, nine of whom carried *Acinetobacter* in previous rectal cultures and two in simultaneous surveillance samples. Lortholary et al. [21] observed that 75% of 96 isolates of *A. baumannii* from 13 infected and 27 colonized ICU patients showed the same genotypic profile, indicating strain identity of colonizing and infecting isolates. Garrouste-Orgeas et al. [23] showed that 91% of ICU-acquired multi-resistant *A. baumannii* and *Klebsiella pneumoniae* infections were preceded by digestive tract colonization. These data are in accordance with results from Corbella et al. [12], who found that 81% of *A. baumannii* infections occurred in ICU patients previously colonized by that microorganism. These investigators were also able to demonstrate strain identity by means of pulsed field gel electrophoresis in isolates from rectal swabs and blood of four patients. Strain identity was also demonstrated by Garrouste-

Orgeas et al. [26], who compared isolates previously present in oropharyngeal swabs with diagnostic isolates of nosocomial pneumonia. Prior oropharyngeal colonization with *A. baumannii* implied a 7.45-fold risk of pneumonia.

Simultaneous environmental sampling has yielded conflicting results. Timsit [11] and Struelens [33] failed to identify exogenous reservoirs. Isolates from the environment were found to be different from those colonizing the respiratory tract and skin of ICU patients in one study [34].

Prevention and Control

Acinetobacter infections persist as a significant problem in many hospitals around the world in spite of intense efforts to implement both standard and exceptional control and prevention measures [11, 12, 20, 35-38]. The existence of occult endogenous reservoirs (human carriage) may, at least in part, account for the difficulty of achieving control and eradication of epidemic outbreaks or endemicity. In fact, clinical diagnostic samples represent only the tip of the iceberg and 50% to 75% of carriers go undetected because they never develop infection [11, 12, 17, 21, 23, 39]. As a result, infection control measures are not initiated and cross-colonization of PPM to other concurrent patients occurs, mainly via the hands of health care workers. In addition, the subset of patients who finally develop infection also are identified late and represent an occult reservoir for a variable time period of colonization [11, 23]. Therefore, surveillance cultures are the indispensable and decisive tool for the design of adequate strategies to control and prevent *Acinetobacter* outbreaks as well as those of other multidrug-resistant microorganisms.

The measures that must be adopted for the prevention and control of *Acinetobacter* colonization and infection in our opinion are self-evident and derive directly from the data exposed above:

Prevention of Spread

Cross-colonization has been shown to occur both during outbreaks and nonoutbreak situations [12, 17, 40-44] and contributes to prolonging or perpetuating colonization and infection. Therefore, handwashing and barrier precautions should be reinforced in order to reduce spread [12, 45]. *Acinetobacter*, however, may extensively contaminate the hospital environment [1], where it is difficult to eradicate [13], and has been reported to survive on dry surfaces for up to 3 weeks [46]. In addition, in the ICU setting 100% compliance with barrier precautions is an unrealistic goal, as has recently been shown by Pittet et al. [47, 48]. In fact, epidemic outbreaks with *Acinetobacter* and other multidrug-resistant microorganisms have repeatedly been refractory to traditional infection control measures [8, 11, 12, 49-52]. Corbella et al. [12], for example, observed that in spite of an intense program of reinforcing of traditional control measures, infections with multi-resistant *A. baumanni* were not significantly reduced. More recently, the same authors [13] report that *A. baumannii* has become endemic in the four ICUs of the hospital and that, one after another, all ICUs had to be closed.

Cross-colonization may be particularly high for *Acinetobacter* for a given colonization pressure [53], i.e., the percentage of patients carrying a PPM, because, compared to vancomycin-resistant enterococci, it is not only present in feces, but also in the upper respiratory tract and skin, and may survive on inanimate surfaces. Bonten et al. [53] recently showed that a colonization pressure of 20% is the main independent risk factor for acquiring vancomycin-resistant *Enteroccus* after admission to the ICU, in spite of high compliance rates with infection control measures. In a previous study, the same investigator [54] had shown that reducing colonization pressure for gram-negative bacilli by applying selective decontamination of the digestive tract (SDD) with oral nonabsorbable antibiotics to half of the patient population of an ICU was associated with significant reductions in colonization and infection.

Eradication of Human Reservoirs

SDD with oral, nonabsorbable antibiotics is aimed at the eradication and prevention of colonization with gram-negative bacteria, *Staphylococcus aureus* (methicillin-sensitive), and yeasts. This simple measure of administering polymyxin E, amphotericin B, and an aminoglycoside, generally tobramycin, every 6 h to the oropharynx (2% paste) and gut (100 mg, 500 mg, and 80 mg, respectively as a 10 ml suspension through the nasogastric tube) is invariably associated with a significant reduction of gram-negative colonization of the gut to a percentage prevalence of approximately 10% [55-58]. Therefore, after it was established that the human digestive tract is the most important epidemiological reservoir for *Acinetobacter* infections, some authors suggested that SDD should be considered in order to reduce carriage [11, 23] and prevent infection. The need for additional interventions is underscored by reports of failure of traditional infection control measures to eradicate colonization and infection with *Acinetobacter* [12, 49], resulting in prolonged outbreaks and endemicity [52]. The existence of multi-resistant or "pan-resistant" strains of *A. baumannii*, only susceptible to polymyxin [4, 59, 60], should be regarded as an additional reason to interrupt the pathophysiologic chain of events that leads to secondary endogenous infections with this microorganism by applying SDD with polymyxin E.

Already 10 years ago, Brun-Buisson et al. [50] demonstrated in a randomized controlled trial that SDD prevented all secondary infections with multi-resistant gram-negative bacilli, mainly *Klebsiella pneumoniae*, and reduced colonization to 3%. No reemergence of colonization or infection was observed during a follow-up period. In a study of a historical control group, Taylor et al. [51] showed the efficacy of administering SDD to all patients admitted for more than 48 h in terminating an outbreak due to *Enterobacter aerogenes*. In both studies SDD was introduced after traditional infection control measures had failed to control the epidemic outbreaks.

SDD trials in which *Acinetobacter* was identified and which report detailed

Table 1. Aerodigestive *Acinetobacter* colonization in SDD trials employing oral polymyxin

Publication	Colonization site	SDD group	Control group	Value
Aerdts et al. [67]	Oropharynx	0 ($n = 17$)	3 ($n = 39$)	
	Stomach	1 ($n = 17$)	4 ($n = 39$)	
Winter et al. [68]	Oropharynx			$p < 0.02$
	Trachea			$p < 0.01$
	Rectum			$p < 0.05$
Ferrer et al. [69]	Stomach	0 ($n = 51$)	4 ($n = 50$)	
	Trachea	1	4	
Verwaest et al. [70]	Tracheobronchial	4 ($n = 220$)	13 ($n = 220$)	
Sánchez García et al. [58]	Tracheobronchial	6 ($n = 131$)	28 ($n = 140$)	$p < 0.05$

Table 2. *Acinetobacter* infections in SDD trials employing oral polymyxin

Publication	Infection	SDD group	Control goup
Ledingham et al. [56]	All secondary	2 ($n = 161$)	5 ($n = 63$)
Ulrich et al. [71]	All, secondary	0 ($n = 52$)	6 ($n = 48$)
Hartenauer et al. [72]	Respiratory tract	0 ($n = 99$)	4 ($n = 101$)
	Sepsis	0	1
Luiten et al. [73]	Pancreatic necrosis	0 ($n = 50$)	3 ($n = 52$)
Winter et al. [68]	Secondary pneumonia	0 ($n = 91$)	2 ($n = 92$)
Korinek et al. [74]	Respiratory tract	1 ($n = 63$)	1 ($n = 60$)
	UTI	2	1
Aerdts et al. [67]	Respiratory tract	0 ($n = 17$)	3 ($n = 39$)
Hammond et al. [57]	All secondary	10 ($n = 114$)	13 ($n = 125$)[a]
Rocha et al. [75]	All secondary	2 ($n = 47$)	15 ($n = 54$)
Total[b]		17/694 (2.4%)	54/734 (7.4%)

[a] Exogenous infections (colonization significantly reduced in SDD group)
[b] CI95 0.03-0.07 $p < 0.01$

microbiologic results of colonization (Tab. 1) and infection (Tab. 2) show lower incidences of *Acinetobacter* in the study groups receiving SDD. The studies were performed during nonoutbreak situations and, therefore, the incidence of *Acinetobacter* reported in the control groups are low and only some studies allow statistical analysis. None of the studies detected increases in the incidence of *Acinetobacter* in the study groups, and no emergence of resistance was reported. The pooled data show a significant reduction of colonization. Infection with *Acinetobacter* is significantly reduced from 7.4% in the control groups to 2.4% in patients receiving SDD.

6. Levin AS, Barone AA, Penco J et al (1999) Intravenous colistin as therapy for nosocomial infections caused by multidrug-resistant Pseudomonas aeruginosa and Acinetobacter baumannii. Clin Infect Dis 28:1008-11

7. Ruiz J, Nunez ML, Perez J et al (1999) Evolution of resistance among clinical isolates of Acinetobacter over a 6-year period. Eur J Clin Microbiol Infect Dis 18:292-529

8. Lyytikainen O, Koljalg S, Harma M, Vuopio VJ (1995) Outbreak caused by two multiresistant Acinetobacter baumannii clones in a burns unit: emergence of resistance to imipenem. J Hosp Infect 31:41-54

9. Wisplinghoff H, Perbix W, Seifert H (1999) Risk factors for nosocomial bloodstream infections due to Acinetobacter baumannii: a case-control study of adult burn patients. Clin Infect Dis 28:59-66.

10. Cisneros JM, Reyes MJ, Pachon J et al (1996) Bacteremia due to Acinetobacter baumannii: epidemiology, clinical findings, and prognostic features. Clin Infect Dis 22:1026-1032

11. Timsit JF, Garrait V, Misset B et al (1993) The digestive tract is a major site for Acinetobacter baumannii colonization in intensive care unit patients. J Infect Dis 168:1336-1337

12. Corbella X, Pujol M, Ayats J et al (1996) Relevance of digestive tract colonization in the epidemiology of nosocomial infections due to multiresistant Acinetobacter baumannii. Clin Infect Dis 23:329-234

13. Corbella X, Pujol M, Argerich MJ et al (1999) Environmental sampling of Acinetobacter baumannii: moistened swabs versus moistened sterile gauze pads [letter]. Infect Control Hosp Epidemiol 20:458-60

14. McDonald LC, Walker M, Carson L et al (1998) Outbreak of Acinetobacter spp. bloodstream infections in a nursery associated with contaminated aerosols and air conditioners. Pediatr Infect Dis J 17:716-722

15. Siau H, Yuen KY, Ho PL et al (1999) Acinetobacter bacteremia in Hong Kong: prospective study and review. Clin Infect Dis 28:26-30

16. Garcia-Garmendia JL, Ortiz-Leyba C, Garnacho-Montero J et al (1999) Mortality and the increase in length of stay attributable to the acquisition of Acinetobacter in critically ill patients. Crit Care Med 27:1794-1799

17. Ayats J, Corbella X, Ardanuy C et al (1997) Epidemiological significance of cutaneous, pharyngeal, and digestive tract colonization by multiresistant Acinetobacter baumannii in ICU patients. J Hosp Infect 37:287-295

18. Garcia-Arata MI, Alarcon T, Lopez-Brea M (1996) Emergence of resistant isolates of Acinetobacter calcoaceticus-A. baumannii complex in a Spanish hospital over a five-year period. Eur J Clin Microbiol Infect Dis 15:512-515

19. Siau H, Yuen KY, Wong SS et al (1996) The epidemiology of acinetobacter infections in Hong Kong. J Med Microbiol 44:340-347

20. Webster CA, Crowe M, Humphreys H, Towner KJ (1998) Surveillance of an adult intensive care unit for long-term persistence of a multi-resistant strain of Acinetobacter baumannii. Eur J Clin Microbiol Infect Dis 17:171-176

21. Lortholary O, Fagon JY, Hoi AB et al (1995) Nosocomial acquisition of multiresistant Acinetobacter baumannii: risk factors and prognosis. Clin Infect Dis 20:790-796

22. Fagon JY, Chastre J, Hance AJ et al (1993) Nosocomial pneumonia in ventilated patients: a cohort study evaluating attributable mortality and hospital stay. Am J Med 94:281-288

23. Garrouste-Orgeas M, Marie O, Rouveau M et al (1996) Secondary carriage with multiresistant Acinetobacter baumannii and Klebsiella pneumoniae in an adult ICU population: relationship with nosocomial infections and mortality. J Hosp Infect 34:279-289

24. Chu YW, Leung CM, Houang ET et al (1999) Skin carriage of acinetobacters in Hong Kong. J Clin Microbiol 37:2962-2967

25. Seifert H, Dijkshoorn L, Gerner-Smidt P et al (1997) Distribution of Acinetobacter species on human skin: comparison of phenotypic and genotypic identification methods. J Clin Microbiol 35:2819-2825

26. Garrouste-Orgeas M, Chevret S, Arlet G et al (1997) Oropharyngeal or gastric colonization and nosocomial pneumonia in adult intensive care unit patients. A prospective study based on genomic DNA analysis. Am J Respir Crit Care Med 156:1647-1655

27. van Saene HK, Damjanovic V, Murray AE, de la Cal MA (1996) How to classify infections in intensive care units-the carrier state, a criterion whose time has come? J Hosp Infect 33:1-12

28. Sánchez M, Mir N, Cantón R et al (1997) The incidence of endogenous gram-positive infections (E-GPI) in critically ill patients (Pts) receiving topical vancomycin (V). A randomized, double-blind, placebo-controlled study. Proceedings of the 37th Interscience Conference on Antimicrobial Agents and Chemotherapy (ICAAC); Toronto [Abstract]

29. Sánchez M, Mir N, Cantón R et al (1997) The effect of topical vancomycin on acquisition, carriage and infection with methicillin-resistant *staphylococcus aureus* in critically ill patients (Pts). A double-blind, randomized, placebo-controlled study. Proceedings of the 37th Interscience Conference on Antimicrobial Agents and Chemotherapy (ICAAC). Toronto, Ontario, Canada [Abstract]

30. Bergmans DC, Bonten MJ, Stobberingh EE et al (1998) Colonization with Pseudomonas aeruginosa in patients developing ventilator-associated pneumonia. Infect Control Hosp Epidemiol 19:853-855

31. Bonten MJ, Hayden MK, Nathan C et al (1996) Epidemiology of colonisation of patients and environment with vancomycin-resistant enterococci. Lancet 348:1615-1619

32. Pittet D, Monod M, Filthuth I et al (1991) Contour-clamped homogeneous electric field gel electrophoresis as a powerful epidemiologic tool in yeast infections. Am J Med 91:256S-263S

33. Struelens MJ, Carlier E, Maes N et al (1993) Nosocomial colonization and infection with multiresistant Acinetobacter baumannii: outbreak delineation using DNA macrorestriction analysis and PCR-fingerprinting. J Hosp Infect 25:15-32

34. Koljalg S, Sults I, Raukas E et al (1999) Distribution of Acinetobacter baumannii in a neurointensive care unit. Scand J Infect Dis 31:145-150

35. Toltzis P, Yamashita T, Vilt L et al (1998) Antibiotic restriction does not alter endemic colonization with resistant gram-negative rods in a pediatric intensive care unit. Crit Care Med 26:1893-1899

36. Goldmann DA, Weinstein RA, Wenzel RP et al (1996) Strategies to prevent and control the emergence and spread of antimicrobial-resistant microorganisms in hospitals. A challenge to hospital leadership. JAMA 275:234-240

37. Shlaes DM, Gerding DN, John JFJ et al (1997) Society for Healthcare Epidemiology of America and Infectious Diseases Society of America Joint Committee on the Prevention of Antimicrobial Resistance: guidelines for the prevention of antimicrobial resistance in hospitals [see comments]. Clin Infect Dis 25:584-99

38. Villers D, Espaze E, Coste-Burel M et al (1998) Nosocomial Acinetobacter baumannii infections: microbiological and clinical epidemiology. Ann Intern Med 129:182-189

39. D'Agata EMC, Venkatraman L, DeGirolami P et al (1999) Colonization with broad-spectrum cephalosporin-resistant Gram-negative bacilli in intensive care units during a nonoutbreak period: prevalence, risk factors, and rate of infection. Crit Care Med 27:1090-1095

40. Husni RN, Goldstein LS, Arroliga AC et al (1999) Risk factors for an outbreak of multi-drug-resistant Acinetobacter nosocomial pneumonia among intubated patients. Chest 115:1378-1382

41. Bergmans DC, Bonten MJ, van Tiel FH et al (1998) Cross-colonisation with Pseudomonas aeruginosa of patients in an intensive care unit. Thorax 53:1053-1058

42. D'Agata EM, Venkataraman L, DeGirolami P, Samore M (1999) Molecular epidemiology of ceftazidime-resistant gram-negative bacilli on inanimate surfaces and their role in cross-transmission during nonoutbreak periods. J Clin Microbiol 37:3065-3067

43. Marques MB, Waites KB, Mangino JE et al (1997) Genotypic investigation of multidrug-resistant Acinetobacter baumannii infections in a medical intensive care unit. J Hosp Infect 37:125-35

44. Arpin C, Coze C, Rogues AM et al (1996) Epidemiological study of an outbreak due to multidrug-resistant Enterobacter aerogenes in a medical intensive care unit. J Clin Microbiol 34:2163-2169

45. Cardoso CL, Pereira HH, Zequim JC, Guilhermetti M (1999) Effectiveness of hand-cleansing agents for removing Acinetobacter baumannii strain from contaminated hands. Am J Infect Control 27:327-331

46. Jawad A, Seifert H, Snelling AM et al (1998) Survival of Acinetobacter baumannii on dry surfaces: comparison of outbreak and sporadic isolates. J Clin Microbiol 36:1938-1941

47. Pittet D, Dharan S, Touveneau S et al (1999) Bacterial contamination of the hands of hospital staff during routine patient care. Arch Intern Med 159:821-826

48. Pittet D, Mourouga P, Perneger TV (1999) Compliance with handwashing in a teaching hospital. Ann Intern Med 130:126-130

49. De Gheldre Y, Maes N, Rost F et al (1997) Molecular epidemiology of an outbreak of multidrug-resistant Enterobacter aerogenes infections and in vivo emergence of imipenem resistance. J Clin Microbiol 35:152-160

50. Brun-Buisson C, Legrand P, Rauss A et al (1989) Intestinal decontamination for control of nosocomial multiresistant gram-negative bacilli. Study of an outbreak in an intensive care unit. Ann Intern Med 110:873-881

51. Taylor ME, Oppenheim BA (1991) Selective decontamination of the gastrointestinal tract as an infection control measure. J Hosp Infect 17:271-278

52. Riley TV, Webb SA, Cadwallader H et al (1996) Outbreak of gentamicin-resistant Acinetobacter baumanii in an intensive care unit: clinical, epidemiological and microbiological features. Pathology 28:359-363

53. Bonten MJ, Slaughter S, Ambergen AW et al (1998) The role of "colonization pressure" in the spread of vancomycin-resistant enterococci: an important infection control variable. Arch Intern Med 158:1127-1132

54. Bonten MJ, Gaillard CA, Johanson WGJ et al (1994) Colonization in patients receiving and not receiving topical antimicrobial prophylaxis. Am J Respir Crit Care Med 150:1332-1340

55. Stoutenbeek CP, van Saene HK, Zandstra DF (1987) The effect of oral non-absorbable antibiotics on the emergence of resistant bacteria in patients in an intensive care unit. J Antimicrob Chemother 19:513-20

56. Ledingham IM, Alcock SR, Eastaway AT et al (1988) Triple regimen of selective decontamination of the digestive tract, systemic cefotaxime, and microbiological surveillance for prevention of acquired infection in intensive care. Lancet 1:785-790

57. Hammond JM, Potgieter PD, Saunders GL, Forder AA (1992) Double-blind study of selective decontamination of the digestive tract in intensive care. Lancet 340:5-9

58. Sánchez García M, Cambronero Galache JA, López Díaz J et al (1998) Effectiveness and cost of selective decontamination of the digestive tract in critically ill intubated patients. A randomized, double-blind, placebo-controlled, multicenter trial. Am J Respir Crit Care Med 158:908-916

59. Cornaglia G, Riccio ML, Mazzariol A et al (1999) Appearance of IMP-1 metallo-beta-lactamase in Europe. Lancet 353:899-900

60. Lopez-Hernandez S, Alarcon T, Lopez-Brea M (1998) Carbapenem resistance mediated by beta-lactamases in clinical isolates of Acinetobacter baumannii in Spain. Eur J Clin Microbiol Infect Dis 17:282-285

61. Brown S, Bantar C, Young HK, Amyes SG (1998) Limitation of Acinetobacter baumannii treatment by plasmid-mediated carbapenemase ARI-2. Lancet 351:186-187 [letter]

62. Kurokawa H, Yagi T, Shibata N et al (1999) Worldwide proliferation of carbapenem-resistant gram-negative bacteria. Lancet 354:955 [letter]

63. Hammond JM, Potgieter PD (1995) Long-term effects of selective decontamination on antimicrobial resistance [see comments]. Crit Care Med 23:637-645

64. Hancock RE (1997) Peptide antibiotics. Lancet 349:418-422

65. Catchpole CR, Andrews JM, Brenwald N, Wise R (1997) A reassessment of the in-vitro activity of colistin sulphomethate sodium. J Antimicrob Chemother 39:255-260

66. Lortholary O, Fagon JY, Buu HA et al (1998) Colonization by Acinetobacter baumanii in intensive-care-unit patients. Infect Control Hosp Epidemiol 19:188-190

67. Aerdts SJ, van Dalen R, Clasener HA et al (1991) Antibiotic prophylaxis of respiratory tract infection in mechanically ventilated patients. A prospective, blinded, randomized trial of the effect of a novel regimen. Chest 100:783-791

68. Winter R, Humphreys H, Pick A et al (1992) A controlled trial of selective decontamination of the digestive tract in intensive care and its effect on nosocomial infection. J Antimicrob Chemother 30:73-87

69. Ferrer M, Torres A, Gonzalez J et al (1994) Utility of selective digestive decontamination in mechanically ventilated patients. Ann Intern Med 120:389-395

70. Verwaest C, Verhaegen J, Ferdinande P et al (1997) Randomized, controlled trial of selective digestive decontamination in 600 mechanically ventilated patients in a multi-disciplinary intensive care unit. Crit Care Med 25:63-71

71. Ulrich C, Harinck-de Weerd JE, Bakker NC et al (1989) Selective decontamination of the digestive tract with norfloxacin in the prevention of ICU-acquired infections: a prospective randomized study. Intensive Care Med 15:424-431

72. Hartenauer U, Thulig B, Lawin P, Fegeler W (1990) Infection surveillance and selective decontamination of the digestive tract (SDD) in critically ill patients-results of a controlled study. Infection 18 [Suppl 1]:S22-S30

73. Luiten EJ, Hop WC, Lange JF, Bruining HA (1995) Controlled clinical trial of selective decontamination for the treatment of severe acute pancreatitis. Ann Surg 222:57-65

74. Korinek AM, Laisne MJ, Nicolas MH et al (1993) Selective decontamination of the digestive tract in neurosurgical intensive care unit patients: a double-blind, randomized, placebo-controlled study. Crit Care Med 21:1466-1473

75. Rocha LA, Martin MJ, Pita S et al (1992) Prevention of nosocomial infection in critically ill patients by selective decontamination of the digestive tract. A randomized, double blind, placebo-controlled study. Intensive Care Med 18:398-404

Chapter 16

An Approach to Controlling *Acinetobacter* Outbreaks in the ICUs

X. Corbella

Introduction

Acinetobacter baumannii has emerged as an important nosocomial pathogen over the last 15 years and hospital outbreaks are increasingly being reported worldwide [1-13]. The genus *Acinetobacter* has undergone many taxonomic changes, making difficult the comparison between historical and modern series. Among the 19 genomic species currently recognized, there are three usually isolated in hospitalized populations: species 2 (*A. baumannii*), 3 and 13 [14-17]. These three species are included in the so-called *A. calcoaceticus-A. baumannii* complex group [18-20]. Nowadays, isolates of *A. baumannii* are almost exclusively hospital-acquired and rarely found in the community [21].

Similarly to other hospital populations, *A. baumannii* commonly causes epidemic infections, which mainly occur in the ICUs. Large outbreaks due to *A. baumannii* have been registered in several countries worldwide [2, 9, 13, 17, 22]. A 6-month survey conducted by Bergogne-Berezin et al. (*Acinetobacter* study group) during 1995-1996 in several hospitals in seven countries (Belgium, France, Germany, Israel, South Africa, Spain, and the United Kingdom) detected that 14% of large institutions had an incidence rate of *Acinetobacter* spp. infections ranging from 5% to >10% [23]. Reported data from a multicenter study of the surveillance of antibiotic resistance in European ICUs (June 1994-June 1995) included 7308 patients from 18 hospitals in Belgium, 40 in France, 20 in Portugal, 30 in Spain, and 10 in Sweden [24]. The study showed that *Acinetobacter* spp. were in 2% of isolates from Belgium, 10% from France, 6% from Portugal, 8% from Spain, and 3% from Sweden. Surveillance of nosocomial infections were also carried out in 30 Spanish ICUs and included data from more than 7000 patients. *Acinetobacter* spp. was the etiologic agent of ventilator-associated pneumonia in 18% of cases in 1994, 10% in 1995 and 13% in 1996. Furthermore, these resistant organisms caused 7% of the primary bacteremia cases in 1996 [25, 26].

Since 1992, a sustained outbreak due to *A. baumannii* has been noted in our 1000-bed tertiary-care teaching institution in Barcelona, Spain, involving more than 1900 patients (60-70% of them during the ICU stay). Currently, this organism constitutes one of the most common causes of nosocomial infection, being the underlying agent in about 20% of ICU infections. Molecular typing procedures showed that endemic isolates pertained to five main clones [12]. Although control measures were repeatedly reinforced during this time, only transitory decreases in the incidence rates of *A. baumannii* were observed following each reinforcement.

Clinical and Microbiological Epidemiology

The hospital epidemiology of *A. baumannii* outbreaks is still only poorly understood, although there is no doubt that both the surprising ability of the genus to acquire antimicrobial multiresistance and its high capacity for survival on most environmental surfaces are determining factors for their spread and persistence in hospitals. Environmental contamination and colonized patients may act as the major epidemiological reservoirs for infection, and inadequate prevention of cross-transmission is the main determinant of its spread and persistence (airborne transmission may play a secondary role). Many contaminated items in the hospital environment have been implicated as the source of infections, and cross-contamination via the hands has been clearly supported by several studies, which documented positive hand and glove cultures from staff members who had been caring for patients [3, 27-29]. Colonized patients may constitute an additional "animate" object of the ICU environment and a continuous reservoir for recontamination of the immediate environment and the hands of healthcare workers. In this way, patients may facillitate the maintenance of the epidemiological cycle of *A. baumannii* infections: environment - staff - patients - staff - environment (Fig. 1).

Nosocomial *A. baumannii* infections are mainly related to the presence of invasive procedures and continuous manipulations or catheters, such as intubation-associated respiratory tract infections, surgical wounds, urinary tract, and primary bacteremia. While *Acinetobacter* spp. have been classically recognized to be of low virulence, some authors have reported high rates of mortality associated with nosocomial pneumonia or bacteremia due to *A. baumannii* [30, 31]. In our experience, morbidity and mortality due to *A. baumannii* is lower than that observed for other hospital-acquired gram-negative bacilli and many *A. baumannii* organisms isolated during admission often reflect colonization rather than infection. Only controlled investigations may determine the true virulence, although they are extremely difficult to conduct since the clinical relevance of isolates is uncertain: they are most often polymicrobial, most occur in severely ill ICU patients, and they are usually associated with multiple invasive procedures.

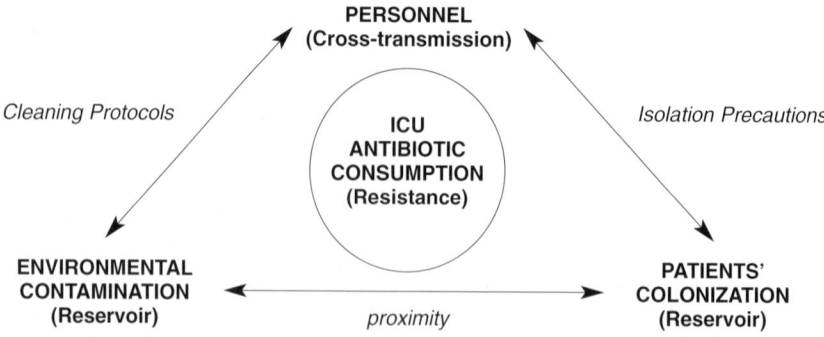

Fig. 1. Epidemiology of *A. baumannii* hospital infections

Molecular typing methods such as pulsed-field gel electrophoresis (PFGE) and polymerase chain reaction (PCR) fingerprinting may contribute to a better epidemiological approach in emerging outbreaks, differentiating endemic from epidemic or sporadic infections. Antibiograms may be of less value when identifying the emergence of *A. baumannii* epidemics since multiresistance is inherent in most current strains isolated worldwide, and unrelated organisms may exhibit the same antibiogram. Furthermore, changes in susceptibility patterns may occur during sustained endemics [8, 11, 32]. Typing studies often show that several clones may be concurrently present during uncontrolled epidemics or sustained endemics by *A. baumannii* [9, 12]. However, a complete correlation between susceptibility pattern and genotyping may be documented in such circumstances [33, 34], facilitating the infection-control management of the outbreak. In any case, molecular typing seems to be required in large outbreaks not only because it is the newest approach, but in order to identify the sources and modes of transmission, and better outline the control strategies for spread prevention [35-37].

An Approach to Controlling *Acinetobacter* Outbreaks

Emerging epidemics by *A. baumannii* limited to a sole ward can usually be eradicated after the identification of a common source of infection and the implementation of basic control measures. Nevertheless, control of large and sustained outbreaks is much more difficult, since a variety of potential sources may be present, making infection-control management a serious challenge. In fact, although no well-defined recommendations have been established yet for such outbreaks, the approach to the outbreak control may include the measures shown in Table 1. Unfortunately, the sequence and priority with which control measures should be applied and the results that physicians might expect are not yet known.

Reinforcement of Isolation Precautions

The cornerstone of control programs in *A. baumannii* outbreaks still lies in handwashing and isolation methods, including the use of protective gloves and gowns. The genus *Acinetobacter* is known to be a normal inhabitant of human skin and several authors have postulated that, in addition to the contaminated environment, patients could be a major reservoir for hospital spread in endemic settings [2, 5, 8-11, 22, 38]. In agreement with this thinking, our group and several other authors showed that not only the skin but also the pharynx, the respiratory tract, and the digestive tract of ICU patients may be colonized by *A. baumannii*, providing permanent carriage and a source for epidemic infections [2, 38-40]. Of relevance was the observation that *A. baumannii* may colonize the digestive tract, since these organisms are not considered to be inhabitants of the bowel in healthy humans [41]. However, it is well-known that in severely ill hospitalized patients, the normal digestive flora which provides intestinal colonization resistance can be modified

Table 1. Recommended control measures in large endemics due to *A. baumannii*

---

1. Cross-transmission prevention
 Prospective screening for colonized patients using body-site swabs
 Cutaneous isolation of patients known to be colonized
 Cohorting patients
 Correct use of gloves and gowns
 Use of cast off or frequent routine spare clothing
 Correct handwashing compliance
 Handwashing facilities in the rooms
 Assigning of an infection-control nurse regarding compliance with measures
 Attention to the use of medical apparatus moved from patient-to-patient
 Attention to movement of colonized patients througout the hospital

2. Environmental decontamination
 Revision of housekeeping practices
 Revision of medical equipment decontamination procedures
 Initial approach to potential environmental sources of infection
 Implementation of a routine surveillance of environmental contamination
 Transitory closing of the ICUs for complete decontamination
 Global redesign of the ICUs

3. Reduction of selective advantage for spread
 Design of antibiotic alternatives for treatment of *A. baumannii* infections
 Antibiotic rotation policies for empirical regimens
 Transitory restriction use of specific antibiotics

4. Reduction of patient reservoir
 Selective intestinal decontamination
 Concomitant digestive, pharyngeal, and cutaneous decontamination

5. Improvement of adequate compliance with control measures
 Educational programs for adequate cross-transmission prevention
 Providing feedback of data referring to rates of contamination
 Providing feedback of data referring to compliance with basic control measures

---

[42], predisposing patients to acquiring persistent colonization by exogenous nosocomial epidemic pathogens.

In our experience, 66% of ICU patients were found to have axillar, pharyngeal, or rectal colonization by *A. baumannii* [33]. Of concern was the surprising speed with which patients were colonized (77% during the first week of ICU stay), and these results agreed with those of other previous reports [8]. Furthermore, at the time of initial detection, more than half of the patients had two or three concomitantly positive body sites, which hampered the identification of a hypothetical sequence of colonization. The probability of remaining free of colonization was less than 25% at 30 days of ICU admission.

When potential risk factors for *A. baumannii* acquisition have been evaluated, terms such as the severity of illness, length of ICU stay, previous days with invasive procedures and, almost uniformly, prior antibiotic administration were found to be the main predisposing conditions, like those reported for other hospital infections [7, 13, 22, 30, 31, 43]. However, when prospective screening for patient colonization was done, we observed that the previous state of an *A. baumannii* carrier was the major attribute for the subsequent development of infections, with regard to those classically associated factors. In fact, this previous carrier state was detected in almost all patients who developed positive clinical samples, with a mean of 7 days between detection of body-site carriage and clinical colonization or infection. Under the special circumstances noted in our ICUs, analysis found those patients submitted to continuous manipulations – such as those with polytrauma, or those who were admitted in an ICU ward with a high "tonnage" of colonized patients – to be at higher risk for body-site colonization.

Since body-site colonization precedes clinical samples (in our setting with a mean of 7 days) in most patients admitted to ICU wards, a surveillance program based on the identification of positive clinical samples may be too late to prevent cross-transmission and the spread of the outbreak. Therefore, in emerging outbreaks, continued prospective screening for colonized patients relying on body-site swabs seems to be mandatory as the initial approach and for early implementation of barrier measures. According to our results, the weekly practice of a single body-site swab (either cutaneous, phryngeal, or rectal) missed fewer than a fourth of the total of colonized patients [33]. From the cost-profit point of view, one should consider whether this miss rate is reasonable or whether in some special circumstances more accurate detection rates by means of a pharyngeal-rectal swab combination (which may detect about 90% of total colonized patients) might be more appropriate.

Unfortunately, appropriate compliance with barrier measures is not always adhered to in a busy ICU (observational studies revealed adequate compliance in only 36-65% of observed opportunities), explaining in part the failure to control *A. baumannii* in endemic settings [44]. Cohorting patients has been shown useful in *A. baumannii* outbreaks as well as in other kind of hospital epidemics [8, 9, 45]. However, in some *A. baumannii* settings, this accumulation of colonized patients could determine a "boomerang" effect, leading to higher rates of environment contamination in those wards if cleaning protocols and cross-transmission prevention are not effectively implemented. Special care should be taken with any medical apparatus such as electrocardiographs or X-rays that are moved daily from patient-to-patient as well as when contaminated patients leave the ICU wards for diagnostic or therapeutic procedures. Furthermore, the fact that the microorganism may survive for several days on clothes used by staff in ICU wards should be taken into account.

Cost-effectiveness and the assumption of the ineluctable advance of increasing rates due to *A. baumannii* and other resistant organisms may be offered by some ICU workers as an excuse for not acting and for decreased compliance with barrier measures. The placing of handwashing facilities in all ICU rooms, the use of disposable clothing or the frequent, routine change of clothing, and assigning an infection-control nurse on the ICUs to provide continuous personnel education, and feedback of data regarding hand carriage and contamination rates might enhance the compliance with basic isolation precautions. Nevertheless, infection-control teams have the ultimate responsibility for reducing cross-transmission and for renewing efforts to maintain infection control programs.

Surveillance of Environmental Contamination and Revision of Cleaning Protocols

It is well known that the ability of the genus *Acinetobacter* to persist on dry surfaces for more than 2 weeks (a time longer than that observed for other gram-negative rods) contributes heavily to the development and persistence of hospital outbreaks. This survival seems to be due to the intrinsic capacity of the organism to survive under different conditions of humidity, temperature, and pH [46-48].

Evaluation of environmental contamination rates in endemic/epidemic settings may differ widely, depending on several factors, such as the magnitude of the outbreak at the time of sampling, the type of items cultured, and the technique used. The overall rates reported for authors ranged between 0% and 18% [10]. Outbreaks affecting a small number of patients can show lower grades of contamination than those which are large and sustained. In addition, the items placed in the immediate environment of a colonized patient may show higher contamination rates. Microbiological techniques used for culturing surfaces may also play a role in such differences. Recommended techniques included Rodac impression agar plates and cotton-tipped swabs moistened with brain heart infusion broth (BHIB). To improve the ability to detect environmental contamination, our group modified the swab technique by using sterile gauze rather than cotton applicator swabs [49].

Routine environmental studies are a useful measure not only to detect the sources of infections, but also to detect potentially unrecognized reservoirs and for monitoring compliance with basic control measures. In this way, we believe that the use of moistened sterile gauze pads probably provides a more sensitive method for sampling. For careful environmental surveillance, items could be grouped as follows:
- Group 1: those belonging to rooms free of patients cultured after terminal cleaning
- Group 2: those placed into an ICU storage room while waiting for new patients
- Group 3: those that are moved daily from patient-to-patient
- Group 4: those placed inside the units and commonly shared by personnel.

Results of environmental surveillance focusing on those groups of items may help identify procedures which are susceptible to improvement and can direct the efforts for appropriate compliance on the part of the personnel responsible. Thus, groups 1, 2, and 3 indicate compliance with housekeeping and cleaning procedures, and group 4 mainly involves compliance with barrier measures and handwashing.

Revision and reinforcement of cleaning protocols should be mandatory when results indicate extensive environmental contamination. Protocols should detail all housekeeping practices and medical equipment decontamination procedures and indicate the schedule as well as the staff responsible for cleaning. Sometimes only temporary closure of the ICUs can assure complete decontamination [1, 32]. In an ICU setting with a high incidence of *A. baumannii*, we repeatedly documented the inability of our cleaning procedures to provide systematic negative cultures in samples obtained from rooms free of patients after terminal cleaning. In contrast, all cultures carried out after the sequential closing, decontaminating, and painting of the ICU wards were found negative. However, efforts to decontaminate the ICUs may unfortunately fail if colonized patients are readmitted after decontamination. This troublesome practice may occur in those tertiary-care public institutions in which the high degree of pressure on medical care and the high density of colonized patients usually determine the rapid recontamination of the ICUs. In endemic settings in which intensive surveillance fails to control the outbreak, other draconian measures such as the structural redesign of the ICUs may be required.

Rational Antibiotic Consumption

Although there is little doubt that antibiotic consumption plays a relevant role in the emergence of resistant organisms in ICUs [50-54], in *A. baumannii* outbreaks, the role of antibiotic use is difficult to establish. These organisms have exhibited one of the most alarming patterns towards antimicrobial resistance over the past two decades, and currently most *A. baumannii* strains isolated worldwide are highly resistant to modern ß-lactams, aminoglycosides, and fluoroquinolones. Under such circumstances exposure to antibiotics may determine a selective advantage for those multiresistant clones over the more susceptible ones [6, 8, 54]. In fact, antibiotic administration has uniformly been reported among the associated risk factors for developing nosocomial infections by the majority of authors [6, 8, 13, 22]. Probably, while strongly insuring strict compliance with basic control measures, antibiotic restriction programs may contribute to containing the spread of antibiotic resistance among the *A. baumannii* population.

Nowadays, the resistance to carbapenems is a matter of great concern, the last recognized antibiotic alternative. Data from the European Surveillance study mentioned above showed carbapenem-resistant strains in 12% of *Acinetobacter* isolates in Belgium, 9% in France, 5% in Portugal, 16% in Spain, and 19% in Sweden [24]. In our hospital, carbapenem resistance emerged and rapidly spread among the *A. baumannii* population in 1997, after 5 years of sustained outbreak. Molecular typing showed that carbapenem resistance was due to the introduction of a new clone colonizing a patient moved from the ICU of another Spanish hospital [54]. Now, in our ICUs, most strains are only sensitive to polymyxins.

In outlining empirical antibiotic schedules it may be very important to know the antibiogram of the *A. baumannii* clones prevailing in each ICU. Because of its low virulence, clinical judgment in selecting which patients really need antibiotics is mandatory. Significantly, some infections may respond to the removal of foreign bodies, débridement, or topical therapy [55] but, in others, multiresistance could make the treatment of infections a challenge for physicians, prompting the use of unusual antibiotics such as sulbactam [8, 56-58].

Selective Intestinal Decontamination

Since the digestive tract was demonstrated to be an important reservoir for *A. baumannii* in ICU patients, some authors have proposed selective decontamination as a measure for control. These optimistic expectations were challenged by two recent studies showing that selective digestive decontamination may not be an effective strategy in preventing *A. baumannii* infections such as nosocomial pneumonia [59, 60]. Possible reasons are the fact that such infections may be exogenous in origin, either from the inanimate environment or from other concomitantly colonized body sites such as the skin or the respiratory tract, probably reflecting the natural habitat for *Acinetobacter* sp. However, it is difficult to state whether both the near environment or the skin could also be contaminated via the extension of the patient's digestive tract colonization. Furthermore, the extremely narrow therapeutic margin shown by the *A. baumannii* population worldwide now casts doubts on the real efficacy of digestive decontamination, since many strains are aminoglycoside resistant (a family of antibiotics usually included in decontamination schedules along with polymyxins).

Conclusions

Taking into account all these reflections, we believe the risk of failure using monotherapy and the potential selection of more resistant *A. baumannii* strains may be reasons for discouraging selective intestinal decontamination in some settings. However, if it is considered, basic infection-control interventions such as strict compliance with cleaning procedures and cross-transmission prevention should be strongly insured, and decontamination should probably not be limited only to the digestive tract, but also to the skin and respiratory tract. Under such circumstances, its hypothetic role in contributing to decreasing secondary environmental contamination and thus increasing the efficacy of other control measures is not known. As the organisms are associated with a low to moderate morbidity, one should consider whether attempts to prevent or eradicate *A. baumannii* infections by implementing body-site decontamination programs is reasonable.

References

1. Sherertz RJ, Sullivan ML (1985) An outbreak of infection with Acinetobacter calcoaceticus in burn patients: contamination of patients' mattresses. J Infect Dis 151:252-258
2. Gerner-Smidt P (1987) Endemic occurrence of Acinetobacter calcoaceticus biovar anitratus in an intensive care unit. J Hosp Infect 10:265-272
3. Hartstein AI, Rashad AL, Liebler JM et al (1988) Multiple intensive care unit outbreak of Acinetobacter calcoaceticus subspecies anitratus respiratory infection and colonization associated with contaminated, reusable ventilator circuits and resucitation bags. Am J Med 85:624-631
4. Sakata H, Fujita K, Maruyama S et al (1989) Acinetobacter calcoaceticus biovar. anitratus septicaemia in a neonatal intensive care unit: epidemiology and control. J Hosp Infect 14:15-22
5. Crombach WHJ, Dijkshoorn L, van Noort-Klaassen M et al (1989) Control of an epidemic spread of a multi-resistant strain of Acinetobacter calcoaceticus in a hospital. Intensive Care Med 15:166-170

6. Buisson Y, Tran van Nhieu G, Ginot L et al (1990) Nosocomial outbreaks due to amikacin-resistant tobramycin-sensitive Acinetobacter species: correlation with amikacin usage. J Hosp Infect 15:83-93

7. Bergogne-Berezin E, Joly-Guillou ML (1991) Hospital infection with Acinetobacter spp.: an increasing problem. J Hosp Infect 18[Suppl A]:250-255

8. Go ES, Urban C, Burns J et al (1994) Clinical and molecular epidemiology of Acinetobacter infections sensitive only to polymyxin B and sulbactam. Lancet 344:1329-1332

9. Seifert H, Boullion B, Schulze A, Pulverer G (1994) Plasmid DNA profiles of Acinetobacter baumannii: clinical application in a complex endemic setting. Infect Control Hosp Epidemiol 15:520-528

10. Bergogne-Berezin E, Towner KJ (1996) Acinetobacter spp. as nosocomial pathogens: microbiological, clinical, and epidemiological features. Clin Microbiol Rev 9:148-165

11. Fang FC, Madinger NE (1996) Resistant nosocomial gram-negative bacillary pathogens: Acinetobacter baumannii, Xanthomonas maltophilia, and Pseudomonas cepacia. Curr Top Infect 16:52-75

12. Dominguez MA, Ayats J, Ardanuy C et al (1998) Evolution and molecular characterization of epidemic clones of multiresistant Acinetobacter baumannii (1992-97). 38th Interscience Conference on Antimicrobial Agents and Chemotherapy. San Diego, Abstract K-124

13. Villers D, Espaze E, Coste-Burel M et al (1998) Nosocomial Acinetobacter baumannii infections: microbiological and clinical epidemiology. Ann Intern Med 129:182-189

14. Tjernberg I, Ursing J (1989) Clinical starins of Acinetobacter classified by DNA-DNA hybridization. Acta Pathol Microbiol Immunol Scand 97:595-605

15. Joly-Guillou ML, Bergogne-Berezin E, Vieu JF (1991) Epidemiology of Acinetobacter strains isolated from nosocomial infections in France. In: Towner KJ, Bergogne-Berezin E, Fewson CA (eds) The biology of Acinetobacter. Plenum, New York, pp 63-68

16. Seifert H, Baginsky R, Schlze A, Pulverer G (1993) The distribution of Acinetobacter species in clinical culture materials. Zentrabl Bakteriol 279:544-552

17. Dijkshoorn L, Aucken HM, Gerner-Smidt P et al (1993) Correlation of typing methods for Acinetobacter isolates from hospital outbreaks. J Clin Microbiol 31:702-705

18. Bouvet PJM, Jeanjean S (1989) Delineation of new proteolytic genospecies in the genus Acinetobacter. Res Microbiol 140:291-299

19. Gerner-Smidt P, Tjernberg I, Ursing J (1991) Reliability of phemotypic tests for identification of Acinetobacter species. J Clin Microbiol 29:277-282

20. Gennari M, Lombardi P (1993) Comparative characterization of Acinetobacter strains isolated from different foods and clinical sources. Zentrabl Bakteriol 279:553-564

21. Joly-Guillou ML, Brun Buisson C (1996) Epidemiology of Acinetobacter spp.: surveillance and management of outbreaks. In: Bergonge-Berezin E, Joly-Guillou ML, Towner KJ (eds) Acinetobacter: microbiology, epidemiology, infections, management. CRC, Boca Raton, pp 73-75

22. Mulin B, Talon D, Viel JF et al (1995) Risk factors for nosocomial colonization with multiresistant Acinetobacter baumannii. Eur J Clin Microbiol Infect Dis 14:569-576

23. Bergogne-Berezin E (1996) Acinetobacter: a challenge to infection control. Acinetobacter 96. Fourth International Symposium on the Biology of Acinetobacter. Eilat, Israel

24. Hanberger H, García Rodríguez JA, Gobernado M et al (1999) Antibiotic susceptibility among aerobic gram-negative bacilli in intensive care units in 5 European countries. JAMA 281:67-71

25. Palomar M, Alvárez Lerma F, de la Cal MA et al (1997) ICU-acquired infections in Spain. Predominant pathogens. Intensive Care Med 23 [Suppl 1]:123

26. Palomar M, Alvárez Lerma F, de la Cal MA et al (1997) Etiología y patrones de sensi-

bilidad de las infecciones adquiridas en los Servicios de Medicina Intensiva. XXXII Congreso Nacional de la Sociedad Española de Medicina Intensiva y Unidades Coronarias (SEMIUC)

27. Patterson JE, Vecchio J, Pantelick EL et al (1991) Association of contaminated gloves with transmission of Acinetobacter calcoaceticus var. anitratus in an intensive care unit. Am J Med 91:479-483

28. Contant J, Kemeny E, Oxley C et al (1990) Investigation of an outbreak of Acinetobacer calcoaceticus var. Anitratus infections in an adult intensive care unit. Am J Inferct Control 18:288-291

29. Corbella X, Montero A, Pujol M et al (2000) Emergence and rapid spread of carbapenem resistance during a large and sustained hospital outbreak of multiresistant acinetobacter baumannii. J Clin Microbiol 38:4086-4095

30. Lortholary O, Fagon JY, Buu-Hoi A et al (1995) Nosocomial acquisition of multiresistant Acinetobacter baumannii: risk factors and prognosis. Clin Infect Dis 20:790-796

31. Kaul R, Burt JA, Cork L et al (1996) Investigation of a multiyear critical care unit outbreak due to relatively drug-sensitive Acinetobacter baumannii: risk factors and attributable mortality. J Infect Dis 174:1279-1287

32. Tankovic J, Legrand P, de Gatines G et al (1994) Characterization of a hospital outbreak of imipenem resistant Acinetobacter baumannii by phenotypic and genotypic typing methods. J Clin Microbiol 32:2677-2681

33. Ayats J, Corbella X, Ardanuy C et al (1997) Epidemiological significance of cutaneous, pharyngeal, and digestive tract colonization by multiresistant Acinetobacter baumannii in ICU patients. J Hosp Infect 37:287-295

34. Vila J, Amela M, Jimenez de Anta MT (1989) Laboratory investigation of hospital outbreak caused by two different multiresistant Acinetobacter calcoaceticus subsp. anitratus strains. J Clin Microbiol 27:1086-1089

35. Vila J, Marcos MA, Jimenez de Anta MT (1996) A comparative study of different typing methods for epidemiological typing of Acinetobacter calcoaceticus-A. baumannii complex. J Med Microbiol 44:482-489

36. Seifert H, Schulze A, Baginsky R, Pulverer G (1994) Comparison of four different typing methods for epidemiological typing of Acinetobacter baumannii. J Clin Microbiol 32:1816-1819

37. Dijkshoorn L (1996) Acinetobacter: Microbiology. In: Bergonge-Berezin E, Joly-Guillou ML, Towner KJ (eds) Acinetobacter: microbiology, epidemiology, infections, management. CRC, Boca Raton, pp 41-64

38. Wise KA, Tosolini FA (1990) Epidemiological surveillance of Acinetobacter species. J Hosp Infect 16:319-329

39. Timsit JF, Garrait V, Misset B et al (1993) The digestive tract is a major site for Acinetobacter baumannii colonization in intensive care unit patients. J Infect Dis 168:1336-1337

40. Corbella X, Pujol M, Ayats J et al (1996) Relevance of digestive tract colonization in the epidemiology of multiresistant Acinetobacter baumannii. Clin Infect Dis 23:329-334

41. Grehn M, von Graevenitz A (1978) Search of Acinetobacter calcoaceticus subsp. anitratus: enrichment of fecal samples. J Clin Microbiol 8:342-343

42. Brun-Buisson C, Legrand P (1994) Can topical and nonabsorbable antimicrobials prevent cross-transmission of resistant strains in ICUs? Infect Control Hosp Epidemiol 15:447-455

43. Seifert H, Strate A, Pulverer G (1995) Nosocomial bacteremia due to Acinetobacter baumannii: clinical features, epidemiology and predictors of mortality. Medicine 74:340-349

44. Wenzel RP, Edmon MB (1998) Vancomycin-resistant Staphylococcus aureus: infection control considerations. Clin Infect Dis 27:245-251

45. French GL, Casewell MW, Roncoroni AJ et al (1980) A hospital outbreak of antibiotic resistant Acinetobacter anitratus: epidemiology and control. J Hosp Infect 1:125-131
46. Getschell-White SI, Donowitz LG, Groschel DHM (1989) The inanimate environment of an intensive care unit as a potential source of nosocomial bacteria: evidence for long survival of Acinetobacter calcoaceticus. Infect Control Hosp Epidemiol 10:402-406
47. Musa EK, Desai N, Casewell MW (1990) The survival of Acinetobacter calcoaceticus inoculated on fingertips and on formica. J Hosp Infect 15:219-227
48. Wendt C, Dietze B, Ruden H (1994) Survival of Acinetobacter species on dry surfaces. Third International Symposium Biology of Acinetobacter. Edinburgh
49. Corbella X, Pujol M, Argerich MJ et al (1999) Environmental sampling of Acinetobacter baumannii: moistened swabs versus moistened sterile gauze pads. Infect Control Hosp Epidemiol 20:458-460
50. Gaynes R (1995) Antibiotic resistance in ICUs: a multifaceted problem requiring a multifaceted solution. Inf Control Hosp Epidemiol 16: 328-330
51. Pallarés R, Pujol M, Peña C et al (1993) Cephalosporins as a risk factor for nosocomial Enterococcus faecalis bacteremia. A matched case-control study. Arch Intern Med 153:1581-1586
52. Peña C, Pujol M, Ardanuy C et al (1998) Epidemiology and successful control of a large outbreak due to Klebsiella pneumoniae producing extended-spectrum ß-lactamases. Antimicrob Agents Chemother 42:53-58
53. Bonten MJ, Hayden MK, Nathan C et al (1996) Epidemiology of colonization of patients and environment with vancomycin-resistant enterococci. Lancet 348:1615-1619
54. Corbella X, Montero A, Pujol M et al (1998) Emergence of carbapenem resistance during a large hospital endemic by multiresistant Acinetobacter baumannii: epidemiology and control measures. The 38th International Conference of Antimicrobial Agent and Chemotherapy (ICAAC), San Diego
55. Viladrich PF, Corbella X, Corral L et al (1999) Successful treatment of carbapenem-resistant Acinetobacter baumannii ventriculitis with intraventricular colistin sulphomethate sodium. Clin Infect Dis 28:916-917
56. Urban C, Go E, Mariano N et al (1993) Effect of sulbactam on infections caused by imipenem-resistant Acinetobacter calcoaceticus biotype anitratus. J Infect Dis 167:448-451
57. Jiménez-Mejías ME, Pachón J, Becerril B et al (1997) Treatment of multi-resistant Acinetobacter baumannii meningitis with ampicillin/sulbactam. Clin Infect Dis 24:932-935
58. Corbella X, Ariza J, Ardanuy C et al (1998) Efficacy of sulbactam alone and in association with ampicillin in nosocomial infections due to Acinetobacter baumannii. J Antimicrobial Chemother 42:793-802
59. Joly-Guillou ML, Wolff M, Decre D et al (1994) Colonization and infection with A. baumannii in ICU patients receiving selective digestive decontamination: results of a case control and molecular epidemiologic investigations. The 34th Interscience Conference on Antimicrobial Agents and Chemotherapy. Orlando, p 103
60. Lance-Sauders G, Hammond JMJ, Potgieter PD et al (1994) Microbiological surveillance during selective decontamination of the digestive tract (SDD). J Antimicrobial Chemother 34:529-544

Chapter 17

Prevention of the Emergence of Resistance

J. Meyer

Introduction

Antimicrobial resistance is a major threat to public health [1]. Multi-resistant microorganisms are not only found in hospitals but also in the community. Infections due to multi-resistant microorganisms cause considerable morbidity and mortality. Thus, the problem of resistant microorganisms is a major problem of public interest [2].

What is Antimicrobial Resistance?

Antimicrobial agents have been developed to control infections. Bacteria are forced to either adapt to antibiotics or to die. Thus, any use (in any dose and over any time period) of antimicrobial agents puts a selective pressure on microbes. Those who survive carry genes for resistance to the antibiotics used. Antimicrobial resistance is not a disease, but rather a natural response of microbes to antibiotics in their environment. In the medical setting, a resistant microbe is one that is not killed by a standard course of antimicrobial treatment. Since half of the antimicrobial agents is used for food production, the development of antimicrobial resistance is not restricted to medical settings.

Bacteria can acquire resistance in a variety of ways [3]. Most of them inherit the genetic information from their predecessors. The replication frequency of bacteria is high. Due to replication errors, genetic mutations occur readily and may spontaneously result in resistance to an antibiotic. Bacteria can also receive genetic material from others possibly carrying the information of antimicrobial resistance. Thus, bacteria are well equiped to develop resistance not only because their ability to multiply rapidly, but also because their exchange of genetic material.

Factors Promoting Emergence
and Spread of Antimicrobial Resistance

Antimicrobial resistance is dependent on both the emergence and spread of resistant microbes. The ability of a microbe to survive a course of antimicrobial therapy can be harmful to the infected patient, since the microbe will multiply and the infection might get worse. Morbidity and mortality due to (resistant) microorganisms is substantial. Epidemiologically, multi-resistant bacteria are transmitted via the hands of health-care providers, to the environment and other patients, in particular in enclosed enviroments such as the ICU.

Emergence of Resistance

The use of antibiotics is a conditio sine qua non for the emergence of antimicrobial resistance [3]. There is increasing evidence that nonmedical use of antibiotics significantly contributes to the emergence of antimicrobial resistance [4]. For example, the introduction of fluoroquinolones in poultry resulted in the emergence of fluoroquinolone-resistant *Campylobacter* sp. Fluoroquinolone-resistant *Campylobacter* infections were not reported before the use of fluoroquinolones in poultry. The glycopeptide avoparcin was used as a growth promoter for more than 30 years. Before 1995, vancomycin-resistant *Enterococcus faecium* could be isolated in more than 80% of broilers. Since the ban of avoparcin in food production in 1995 in Denmark and EU-wide in 1997, the incidence of vancomycin-resistant *E. faecium* in broilers is steadily decreasing and was less than 10% in 1998. However, despite the ban of avoparcin, antibiotics are still used as growth promoters and related to the emergence of resistance. The use of streptogramins in poultry is associated with resistance to these agents in poultry. A combination of two streptogramins (quinupristin and dalfopristin) is used in the therapy of life-threatening infections with otherwise resistant gram-positive bacteria, mainly methicillin-resistant *Staphylococcus aureus* (MRSA) and vancomycin-resistant *Enterococcus* sp (VRE).

Similarly, the use of antimicrobial agents in humans readily led to antibiotic resistance in clinical isolates from patients, in particular those admitted to hospitals and especially intensive care and high dependency units. Data from the United States National Nosocomial Infections Surveillance System (NNIS) showed that the percentage of resistant microorganisms was higher in hospitals than in outpatient isolates [5]. ICU isolates showed a higher incidence of antimicrobial resistance than isolates from general units. In Europe, the average MRSA rate found in ICU isolates was 60%, the highest prevalence was found in Italy (81%) and France (78%) [6]. Resistance of Pseudomonas aeruginosa isolates to gentamicin, imipenem, ceftazidime, and ciprofloxacin was 46%, 21%, 28%, and 26%, respectively [6].

Spread of Resistance

Transmission is the most important factor promoting spread of resistance. Particularly in ICU environments, failure of barrier precautions may be due to the urgent nature of some critical care procedures. In addition, the incidence of infection in ICU patients is high. This is due to the immuno paralysis in the critically ill. Many ICU patients have one or more indwelling devices such as intravascular catheters, endotracheal tubes, and drains compromising normal skin and mucosal barrier functions. As a result, critically ill patients have a high incidence of infections requiring antimicrobial therapy. In a prevalence study performed in 1992, 62% of the patients received antibiotics for therapy or prophylaxis [6].

Nosocomial infections contribute to mortality, morbidity, and costs. Therefore, evidence-based infection prevention guidelines have been developed [7, 8]. However, failure to follow these guidelines contributes to increased infections rates and transmission of resistant pathogens.

Surveillance of Resistance

Surveillance of bacterial resistance is regarded as a key element in the understanding of the problem of resistance [9]. Since antimicrobial resistance is a global threat, nationwide surveillance systems are expected to coordinate information gathered by local committees and laboratories. The European Union has funded the establishment of the European Antimicrobial Resistance Surveillance System (EARSS), located in the Netherlands (http://www.earss.rivm.nl). EARSS has been designed to collect comparable and quantitative data concerning antimicrobial resistance and will cooperate with other organizations involved in WHO networks. EARSS started in April 1998 with an 18-month pilot study on *Streptococcus pneumoniae* and *Staphylococcus aureus*.

Limiting the Factors Promoting Antimicrobial Resistance

Minimizing Emergence of Resistance

Since antimicrobial use is one of the most important factors in the emergence of antimicrobial resistance, prudent use of antibiotics is a cornerstone in the prevention of resistance. A rational use of antimicrobial drugs is dependent on educated staff and surveillance of antibiotic use. For example, the Hospital Infection Control Practices Advisory Committee (HICPAC) of the CDC has published guidelines for the prudent use of vancomycin [10] (see Tables 1, 2).

Antimicrobial use for the treatment of infections should be done with the most effective, least toxic, and – ideally – least expensive drug for the precise duration needed to prevent reoccurrence of infection (Table 3). Optimal antimicrobial therapy often requires cooperation of the intensive care specialist and the infectious disease specialist or microbiologist. Development of local guidelines and treatment algorithms is dependent on knowledge of both the local microbial environment and specific characteristics of the patient population being treated. For example, a trauma ICU will be confronted with infections different than those found on a coronary care unit. A second step to optimize antimicrobial therapy might be the selective removal or restricted use of specific agents. Compliance with restriction

Table 1. Vancomycin is appropriate or acceptable (modified from [10])

- Serious infections caused by betalactam-resistant gram-positive bacteria
- Infection caused by gram-positive bacteria in patient with allergy to beta-lactam antibiotics
- Antibiotic-associated colitis, which is life-threatening or unresponsive to metronidazole treatment
- Endocarditis prophylaxis according to recommended guidelines
- Surgical wound prophylaxis in procedures involving implants or devices in institutions with a high rate of infections caused by MRSA or MRSE. Prophylaxis should be discontinued after a maximum of two doses

Table 2. Vancomycin use should be discouraged (modified from [10])

- Routine surgical prophylaxis other than in patients with life-threatening allergy to betalactam antibiotics
- Empiric antibiotic therapy for a febrile neutropenic patient, unless there is evidence for an infection caused by gram-positive bacteria (e.g., contaminated Hickman catheter) and a high prevalence of infection due to MRSA
- Treatment as a response to a single blood culture for coagulase-negative *staphylococcus*, if other blood cultures taken during the same time frame are negative
- Systemic or local prophylaxis for infection or colonization of indwelling vascular devices
- As part of selective digestive decontamination
- En order to eradicate MRSA
- Primary treatment of antibiotic-associated colitis

Table 3. Proposed methods to control antimicrobial use according to [11]

- Optimal use of antibiotics
- Restriction policies for specific agents
- Cyclic or rotational use
- Combination therapy

policies can be easily controlled and have been partly shown to be effective [11]. A third method proposed is cyclic or rotational antimicrobial use. However, this recommendation has not yet been sufficiently substantiated by clinical trials. The same is true for combination antimicrobial therapy. Although theoretically attractive and already practiced for the treatment of critically ill patients, controlled clinical trials assessing combination therapy are needed [11].

Minimizing Spread of Resistance

As already indicated above, a major factor in the fight against bacterial resistance is the compliance with infection prevention protocols. However, at the administrative level, compliance with recommend prevention measures has been reported to be poor [12]. In 1990, only a minority of ICUs (31%) had written instructions implementing current infection prevention guidelines. Compliance with all recommended practice was 31% for prevention of pneumonia, 22% for prevention of intravascular device-associated infections, and 40% for prevention of urinary tract infection [12].

In addittion, the incidence of individual failure to follow basic hygiene measures is high. The by far most important single measure, the hand disinfection with alcohol-based solutions (or hand washing with antiseptic soaps in the US) is only done properly in the minority of cases. For example, average compliance with hand washing was 48% in a recent published observational study [13], consistent with earlier publications [14, 15]. Disturbingly, noncompliance was especially high among physicians, despite the knowledge that good compliance with hand washing may result in reduced morbidity [16, 17]. Low compliance with handwashing is due to the high workload [13] and may explain why spread of resistant pathogens has not been effectively controlled despite appropriate written infection control policies [18, 19]. It has been acknowledged that health-care workers failed to fully understand the importance of hand disinfection [18]. This failure is hypothesized to reflect fundamental attitudes, beliefs and behaviors, so that simple and quick solutions are not to be expected.

Improvement of hand washing requires ongoing education and control. Further, it is vital to comply with current prevention standards. It is not the lack of data or recommendations but the failure to comply with the existing standards that contributes to transmission of resistant pathogens.

Isolation Precautions

Since the main mode of transmission of resistant microorganisms (especially MRSA) is via hands which become contaminated by contact with colonized or infected patients, application of isolation procedures is essential to minimize transmission of resistant microorganisms. The HICPAC has defined different levels of isolation precautions. Implementation of "standard precautions" is regarded as the primary strategy for successful nosocomial infection control. Standard precautions include:
- Hand washing/hand disinfection after touching blood, body fluids, and contaminated items, whether or not gloves are worn
- Wearing gloves when touching blood, body fluids, and contaminated items
- Wearing mask, eye protection, and face shield to protect eyes, nose, and mouth during procedures that are likely to generate splashes or sprays of blood and body fluids
- Wearing a gown to protect skin and to prevent soiling of clothing during procedures that are likely to generate splashes or sprays of blood and body fluids.

Once a patient is known to be colonized or infected with a resistant microbe, measures to control spreading of this resistant strain are required. Patients with an increased risk of carriage of multi-drug resistant microorganisms should undergo "contact precautions". In addition to standard precautions, contact precautions include:
- Patient placement in a private room or cohorting
- Wearing gloves when entering the room
- Wearing a gown when entering the room and substantial contact to patient or items has to be anticipated
- Limiting the movement and transport of the patient from the room to essential purposes only
- Dedicating patient-care equipment (e.g., stethoscope) to a single patient whenever possible. Equipment, which has to be used on multiple patients, must be adequately cleaned and disinfected before use on another patient.

Selective Digestive Decontamination

The strategy of selective decontamination (SDD) was originally designed not to control resistance but to prevent nosocomial pneumonia. Based on the observation that most nosocomial pneumonias are secondary endogenous, i.e., the patient acquires a microbe in the hospital and gets colonized in the gastrointestinal tract before he/she gets infected, SDD aims at the eradication of potentially pathogenic microbes form the gastrointestinal tract by applying topical antibiotics, by a high standard of infection control practices, by microbial surveillance of the gastrointestinal tract (oral and rectal swabs), and by a course of cefotaxim to treat / prevent primary endogenous infection. Thus, some elements of the SDD protocol and of the guidelines for the prevention of microbial resistance are similar. This is especially true for a high standard of hygiene and for microbial surveillance. SDD significantly reduces morbidity and mortality [20, 21]. Since the introduction of SDD there has been understandable concern that SDD may promote antimicrobial resistance. Current data do not support these concerns, since no significant problems with resistance resulting from SDD usage have been reported [22]. Strict surveillance leads to early identification of patients colonized with resistant microbes. Once the emergence of resistance has been recognized, spread of the resistant strain can be effectively prevented by isolation precautions and other measures. If microbes resistant to SDD agents are detected, the SDD protocol has to be adapted or withdrawn in this individual patient. However, emergence during prophylaxis with SDD is a rare event. In our institution (three ICUs with a total of 25 beds), the full SDD protocol has been implemented since 1990. Resistance was studied in details between 1995 and 1997. Resistance among aerobic gram-negative bacilli was initially absent. Seven patients carried MRSA on admission. Topical vancomycin cleared MRSA carriage, and VRE was not diagnosed. In our institution a decade of SDD has not been associated with emergence of resistance. Therefore, one might speculate that the SDD protocol not only decreases mortality and morbidity due to nosocomial pneumonia but also may contribute to the prevention of emergence of resistance.

References

1. Wise R, Hart T, Cars O, et al (1998) Antimicrobial resistance. Is a major threat to public health. BMJ 317:609-610
2. Fidler DP (1998) Legal issues associated with antimicrobial drug resistance. Emerg Infect Dis 4:169-177
3. Levy SB (1998) The challenge of antibiotic resistance. Sci Am 278:46-53
4. Wegener HC, Aarestrup FM, Jensen LB et al (1999) Use of antimicrobial growth promoters in food animals and Enterococcus faecium resistance to therapeutic antimicrobial drugs in Europe. Emerg Infect Dis 5:329-335
5. Fridkin SK, Gaynes RP (1999) Antimicrobial resistance in intensive care units. Clin Chest Med 20:303-316
6. Vincent JL, Bihari DJ, Suter PM et al (1995) The prevalence of nosocomial infection in intensive care units in Europe. Results of the European Prevalence of Infection in Intensive Care (EPIC) Study. EPIC International Advisory Committee. JAMA 274:639-644.

Main Symbols

AG NB	Aerobic Gram-negative bacilli
APACHE-II	Acute physiology and cronic health evaluation II
BAL	Bronchoalveolar lavage
BHIB	Brain heart infusion broth
BT	Bacterial translocation
CAA	Clinically appropriate antibiotics
CAP	Community-acquired pneumonia
CNS	Coagulase-negative staphylococci
CRBI	Catheter-related bloodstream infections
GIT	Gastrointestinal tract
GNB	Gram-negative bacilli
HAP	Hospital acquired pneumonia
HCW	Health care worker
ICO	Intracellular organisms
IPI	Intrinsic pathogenicity index
ITU	Intensive therapy unit
LOS	Length of stay
MDR	Multiply drug-resistant
MOF	Multiple organ failure
MSSA	Methicillin-sensitive Staphylococcus aureus
MRSA	Methicillin-resistant Staphylococcus aureus
PBPs	Penicillin-binding proteins
PFGE	Pulsed-field gel eletrophoresis
PNI	Prognostic nutritional index
PPM	Potentially pathogenic microorganisms
PRISM	Pediatric risk of mortality
PSB	Protected specimen brush
PTA	Polymyxin E, tobramycin, amphotericin B
SDD	Selective decomination of thedigestive tract
SSSI	Skin and skin structure infections
TEN	Total enteral nutrition
TPN	Total parenteral nutrition
VAP	Ventilator associated pneumonia
VRE	Vancomycin-resistant enterococci